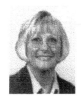

Dear Reader:

Whether you've had a stroke or are a Caregiver, I hope that this book has given you some beneficial information.

If you wish to contact me personally, I would be delighted chat with you.

Marty O. Hopps, Psy.D. (949) 855-0807

A donation o

f $10 would be appreciated to help defray costs of distribution, please send to:

5083 Ovalo, Laguna Woods CA 92653

Post-Stroke Hope

A Motivational Journey to Recovery

POST-STROKE HOPE

A Motivational Journey to Recovery

Marty O. Hopps, Psy.D.

Rutledge Books, Inc.

Danbury, CT

Rutledge Books, Inc.
107 Mill Plain Road, Danbury, CT 06811
1-800-278-8533
www.rutledgebooks.com
info@rutledgebooks.com

Manufactured in the United States of America

Cataloging in Publication Data
Hopps, Marty O., 1937-
    Post-stroke hope

    ISBN: 1-887750-88-6

    1. Cerebrovascular disease -- Patients -- Rehabilitation.
    2. Cerebrovascular Disorders -- rehabilitation -- personal
narratives.
    I. Title.

616-81   98-65859

Dedication

To my blended family:

First my children, Randy and Jennifer;
And to their children Jessica, Samantha, Martina.
May my descendants learn from my lessons in life.

Second, to my stepchildren, Kevin, Shaun, J'me;
And to their children, Ian, Parker, Adam, Markay, Norman and Megan, as well as all their mates, Rosalia, Ray, Robin, Laurie, Tom. And not forgetting, Gillian and Ben, Uncle Tony, and our friend, father, grandfather, great-grandfather, Oliver.
Your sturdy support is what I needed most and am truly thankful.

And, to Mary, my loving, talented, sensitive sister, whose cheerful spirit throughout our lives has given me reason to christen her "Merry."

But most of all, to my husband Norm, whose persistent patience and unexpected new challenge in life as caregiver have surpassed all notions of constant unconditional love. Through his dedicated devotion, permanent patience, humor, style, and smile, I have accepted growth and healing. His hand has replaced the one I have [temporarily] lost, giving me reason to salute my most treasured word — HOPE.

To all the stroke survivors and their families who are learning wisdom from their fate, remember: even though healing from stroke may be your challenge, the real test, the true gift is the triumph of human spirit — HOPE. Follow me and I will show the way...

Tribute

TWO DAYS PRIOR TO RECEIVING THE GALLEYS FOR THIS BOOK, I HAD A PHONE call from my friend, Jackie. She told me she saw Dale Evans on a television show promoting her book, *A Stroke of Hope*, written apparently about *her* stroke. While I have not experienced being a celebrity, needless to say, my first reaction was disappointment: due to the similarity of our book titles. I had worked too long and hard for my title to be in a vying position with someone else's, albeit a celebrity. A few days following this announcement I thought, Why not?! Why not give a tribute to Dale Evans. She has been an archetype in my consciousness since I was a child; and, strokes affect every survivor differently — celebrity or non-celebrity; thus, I began feeling the spirit of the universe touching me gently with love. Instantly, I blessed Dale Evans' title, as well as mine, having personally experienced the reality of hope following a stroke.

Consequently, this tribute is for Dale Evans, as well as all those who have painfully shared their stroke sorrow silently, without adequate words to amplify their inner world of wanting, needing to express their notion hope.

My personal story cries out to everyone who is witness to this condition who may wish to promote their own story as well. Knowing, coping, and hoping are the key words for recovery. Therefore, my story was written with compassion for all the silent stroke survivors who are unknown soldiers of hope.

Acknowledgments

RESEMBLING A MULTI-COLORED TAPESTRY, THE PEOPLE MENTIONED IN THIS journey are many, and I am grateful they wove such colorful threads on this enlightened path. The team at my Western American University — specifically Drs. Bonnie Price, Robert Morrison, Jon Rich, Gary Miller was essential in completing this life design of healing. Richard and angel Pat Koeth: I thank you as well. My medical support at the beginning and during this journey was most important and needed, offering more than medicine: Drs. King, Sethi, Summit, O'Carroll, Hammit, Pearson, Gittleman, Milchiker, Silvers, and Grossman all contributed to my feeling of healing.

My friends are many. Indeed, so many if all were mentioned, it would clutter this section like knots caught on canvas. In the hospital, the two Michaels, resembling distinguished, appointed angels appearing from heaven on a cloudy day, spoke gently about tomorrow radiating sunshine. Everyone's smiles and support have given me the meaning of shared friendship on this journey. An example: Phyllis, you led the way. Weekly Attitudinal Healing members are continually sensitive to my current needs; and I appreciate our powerful healing circle of love. Jean and Soupy, your soul and suggestions were the frame on this tapestry. It sparkles because of you.

My editor, Ida Wood and her eagle eyes, were responsible for carrying me over the threshold into the world of words onto the page. Opening the door was Carol Paradis-Harris who collaborated with wisdom and care in the initial proposal process; whose suggestions I am thankful I followed. Karen Herb and her creative revisions took my story from the halls of researched academia into the realm of universal readership. Because of her talents my joy in recovery reflects the message: HOPE. Rutledge Books, and their discerning team of experts manifested magic in producing this package, which I am proud to accept, and acknowledge as another healing miracle.

Over the threshold, through the door, near to the hearth, close to my heart is my family: the sturdy brace needed for recovery. They know who they are. We are an authentic bunch of the blended stuff: a recipe with us that works. I hug each one for their belief in my being healed. This goes beyond the printed page.

Last and lovingly to my husband Norm: to his smile, his hope, his hand, replacing the one I lost. Can you feel my three hand squeezes saying, I love you?

Dr. Marty O. Hopps

Contents

Foreword

DEALING WITH ILLNESS IS MUCH LIKE WRESTLING WITH AN ANGEL. IN THE BIBLE, the patriarch Jacob returns home to confront the dark-troubled past deeds and deceits of his brother Esau. On the eve of this confrontation, Jacob dreams of wrestling with an angel of God. Jacob would not let go of the angel until he extracted a blessing for himself and his children, but in the process he is permanently injured. He must always walk with a limp, but he is so transformed on the inner levels that his name is changed to Israel — He who struggles with God.

Marty's story of her stroke — her long disability and gradual recovery — is a parallel story for all who struggle with illness. Each person's struggle with illness is their own struggle with the angel of God. The possibilities of transformation are great, while the pain and suffering may seem overwhelming. Holding on to extract the blessing within the illness is the key to this process. Marty shares her path of this process. It is inspiring and filled with wisdom.

As a family physician of over 20 years, I have seen many people wrestle with illness. Some have made remarkable recoveries and inspire others with their love, courage and tenacity. Some become depressed and withdraw from the world. Some never recover, but inspire others in the process of passing on from this world.

Marty has been a part of my weekly attitudinal-healing group for several years. She has inspired me as I have watched the process of wrestling with her stroke. I have seen her love, her strength, and her pain and struggle. I have learned much from Marty.

While we don't seem to have a choice of our illness, we do have freedom to choose our attitude toward the illness. Please read this book and let Marty's story give you strength to wrestle with the angel God has sent you.

Michael Grossman, M.D.
Director of Attitudinal Healing Center of El Toro
Director of Wellness Center of El Toro

Prologue

IT WAS A PEACEFUL NOVEMBER SUNDAY AFTERNOON. THE WEATHER WAS unusually hot outside. Weather forecasters said it was almost a record. I sat in my cream-colored leather and brass chair at my glass dining room table. My Post-Stroke Hope manuscript rested in a pile, like scattered autumn leaves, on top of the recently cleansed table top. Husband Norm was sneaking a nap on the pastel couch in the den next to me. He was snoring slightly.

My plan was to assemble my manuscript pages with brads in order to send it to my new literary agent. The box of brads was opened. With only my right hand — my only functioning hand — I took the three-holed pages and tried to tap them together on the table making a neat pile that would easily accept the three brads. Tap, tap tap. Trying to tap softly so as not to awaken Norm was my objective. He deserves to have his Sunday nap, I thought. He continued to snore softly. Good, my mind said. I was able to secure a couple of stacks of pages lined up evenly, the three holes aligning. Now to put in the brads. With my fumbling right hand eager to insert them, I tried and failed. I tried again. No success.

"Damn," I said to myself, speaking softly under my breath. "I can't insert these into the holes with one hand. It's impossible."

What to do? Impulsive as usual, wanting this to be done immediately, I closed my eyes, feeling frustrated at not being able to do the job myself. All I could do was patiently wait for Norm to awaken from his Sunday nap. How unfair, I thought, having to ask him again for his help. I tried counting to ten with my eyes closed and waited for Norm to open his.

At last he opened his sleepy blue eyes and I approached him with the task of the moment. Within seconds he inserted the brads without a whimper. I'm so fortunate to have him, I told him again. He always helps me so much. I also told him I wished I could do things like that myself, being envious of two-handed people. Norm already knew this, because I had told him often.

When my eyes were closed while Norm was napping and I was tapping, I reflected back on the reason for my clumsy, paralyzed left hand and left side. Some may wonder why. The reason was from my stroke. A stroke at age 48 - from heart bypass surgery during the post-operative period while in the Intensive Care Unit.

The manuscript I was attempting to assemble was my dissertation from my Doctor of Psychology degree. The manuscript, made into book form, is what follows. It is my stroke story.

My university instructors allowed me to write my stroke journey in a "retroflective" narrative format. It became my final dissertation. The first draft was basically my personal stroke journey with Norm and myself as the main characters. Resembling a love story, some remarked, it included all of the torture and hard work I went through during my rehabilitation. It spoke of my fears, my tears, the feelings of helplessness, loss of control, hopelessness. It reflected how I thought my fulfilling life was over. A disaster. A terrible tragedy. It also chronicled the progress I'd made, the setbacks, the personal agony I felt in and out of the hospitals. The meaning of family, friends and supporters was also included. Devastating isolation, darkness, depression, and demons revealed that a darker cauldron was smoldering at the core. A brighter edge evolved, eventually. A spiritual, sensitive side could not be ignored. I spoke about my father's death as a young child, the meaning of my loss, and what it meant to be a woman at my age in this culture, at this time of my mature life. It was an honest medley of feelings from the standpoint of a wounded animal — a snapshot of a female's struggle to regain her wholeness, wholeness of being as an independent person.

The university instructors told me this draft was unacceptable. It was not scholarly. I was required to include much more research. Therefore, I went back to the University of California, at Irvine (UCI) library and scouted thoroughly for the latest information and facts on stroke.

There was one major problem. I could not lift, carry, or copy — with one hand — the huge, heavy bound journals and volumes. I needed Norm's help . . . again.

Weekend after weekend we went to the modern library, Norm helping to lift, carry and copy the multitude of volumes of material. I sifted, sorted, resorted, and went back to my computer, typing with one hand what you are about to read. Huge paper mountains soon became my completed manuscript. Now it contained a love story with research paralleling it, like loving rhymes on valentines.

My purpose is to help others who have had a similar devastating stroke affecting their minds, their bodies. I wanted this material to be meaningful to their caregivers and friends as well. I thought perhaps those in the healing, helping professions would benefit in addition, learning directly from a stroke survivor.

Recently, while working in a care facility as a part of my internship hours, I came upon a rude, abrupt awakening: I was not able to use a clipboard with one hand — a necessary tool in my clinical practice. Horrified, I left the building realizing, still after 11 years, I am newly challenged each day by tasks that a one-handed stroke survivor just can't do. But there are other things I can do and enjoy doing. One is reflecting. Another is writing — with one hand — and working with people. That clipboard experience taught me that perhaps there is something glorious ahead on my path that means my mission is still in the making — an inspired creation in the hands of God. Otherwise, I would have been able to use that clipboard. A lesson? Perhaps.

It is my aim to construct my story as it flows from my fingertips, as the spirit flows from my soul, on an unconscious level, teaching, reaching those who can benefit from my stroke story. In essence, conceivably this havoc will be turned around into pillars of powerful, positive, shimmering glimmers of hope, like a mighty miracle or a rainbow after a storm. Follow me as I reflect, write, teach.

Preface

**. . . Perhaps this havoc has been my intermission
from my mission. . . .**

THIS DOCUMENTATION OF MY PERSONAL JOURNEY, RECOVERING FROM A STROKE
that occurred during heart bypass surgery when I was age 48, will
reflect the arduous task of recovery (a process still pending) with
the intent of offering instant insight to those who have suffered
this personal assault, and to the families, as well as to those in the
helping professions who could gain from this anecdotal account,
serving as a helpful, hopeful, motivational, and perhaps inspirational testimony that says: "yes, there is life after a stroke," which
can be shared with others who are at the beginning of this sometimes frightening journey.

The goal is to tell the story from the beginning as it happened,
in simple terms, progressing to the point where I am now.
Demonstrating recovery is a process — as most things are — and
by admitting my anger, frustration, denial, naiveté, yet showing
tenacity guided by my inner faith, I can continue to conquer the
devastating destruction of body and mind that a stroke delivers,
substantiating the fact that there is definitely post-stroke hope.

Even though it is a simple story, its pathos and passion are real, as was my perseverance. It involves many people whose own personal lives are affected — sometimes subtly, sometimes substantially — forever, mirroring the magic of love that usually heals most wounded animals, like a mighty miracle, or a rainbow after a storm.

This book is a 10-year retroflective narrative — beginning with a personal, brief history, acquainting the reader with pre-stroke material, leading up to the actual event, followed by the post-stroke path.

The past data is necessary to establish what I refer to as "B.S.": Before Stroke behavior. (See the three photographs in the conclusion: one as I looked B.S., one after the stroke while in the hospital, and the last one as I appeared recently. From these visuals, one can estimate the quality of life during these periods). I support this by a written account depicting the degree of what I thought and felt. Feelings are the most valuable to acknowledge in my healing process.

Augmenting my documentation is current stroke information and stroke statistics mainly from The American Heart/National Stroke Association literature, as the research reviewed revealed this data is the most current.

Psychological implications will describe the multifactor healing process, entwined with goals, plans, procedures and techniques that allow healing and recovery.

My personal retroflective narrative amplifies my conscious connection with my unconscious: writing "as the spirit flows from my soul," similar in style to C.G. Jung's autobiography, *Memories, Dreams, Reflections* and J. Bolene's *The Tao of Psychology*. This "stream of consciousness" maps my journey from my heart to paper, expressing how my life changed in an instant.

Within this basic structure acting as an adhesive, I have included research findings that uphold my personal journey. For the benefit of easier reading, I created a "Technical Appendix" for anyone who is interested in addressing this subject in a more in-depth manner. I have also retained the bibliography from my dissertation for further reference.

Several pieces of my research bear special mention. An informative article[1] documented stroke case studies reported in a journalistic style, creating clarity for the average person in an already difficult to understand field. The book *Can You Hear the Clapping of One Hand?* by Veith offers comforting anecdotal accounts, along with informative experiential education, in a sensitive, instructive style.

Anyone who is astute in the commercial world to scientific subjects (otherwise difficult to understand, albeit made easy to comprehend by journalistic anecdotes) can view reports on bestseller lists generating information . . . and controversy. Refer to the Bibliography under Kramer, Brogan, Shriller and Bennett (recently seen on ABC's Prime Time Live news magazine).

Thus, having reformatted my original dissertation into a clear journalistic style, easy for the average reader to understand, the questions to be answered within this book are: What exactly is a stroke? What factors influence stroke recovery? What is the subjective experience of recovery from stroke? Is there life following stroke? If so, what is the predicted quality? What can be expected in treatment following onset of stroke? Is there post-stroke hope? How are friends and family important? What are some stroke statistics?

---

[1] See Calvanio and Levine in the Bibliography for a complete citation.

stroke statistics[2]

Stroke is the nation's most neglected health problem. Given stroke's tremendous impact on Americans, it doesn't receive the attention it deserves.

1. Stroke strikes 550,000 Americans every year.

2. Stroke kills 150,000 Americans annually.

3. Stroke is the most common cause of disability in American adults, robbing them of their most productive years.

4. Stroke is one of our country's most expensive medical problems. Stroke costs our nation $30 billion annually, including hospitalization, physician services, rehabilitation services, nursing homes, and medical equipment such as wheelchairs.

5. Indirect costs, such as lost productivity, total $13 billion per year.

6. The average cost per patient during the first 90 days following a stroke is $15,000.

7. Despite the costs and effects, the public remains uninformed about stroke, especially stroke symptoms and prevention.

8. Why is stroke so neglected? Most likely, it is because of inaccurate but deep-seated misperceptions about the nature of stroke (National Stroke Association, 1994).

Let the curtain of mystery rise, and my narrative commence.

---

[2] National Stroke Association literature, 1994. See the Appendix for address and phone number to contact the National Stroke Association.

Introduction

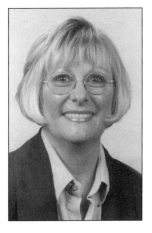

HAVE YOU EVER THOUGHT ABOUT TRYING — with one hand — to do the following? Tie your shoelaces; button a blouse; cut a hangnail; stuff, address, or open an envelope; tear a stamp from a sheet; style your hair with a curling iron; cut meat; butter a roll; use a can opener; eat a hamburger; take care of personal, feminine needs; iron; wrap a package; fold laundry; sew on a button or fix a rip; change the bed linens; change a baby's diaper, pick up and hold a baby; or type this book.

These are just a few challenges to someone who becomes paralyzed on one side, or who has incapacitated one arm. Those who have broken an arm know. It was through trial and error, adjusting, readjusting, and finally acceptances, that I have learned how to adjust to my [temporary] handicap of having a stroke during bypass surgery when I was 48.

I am now in my tenth year of acceptance. The stroke date was a day of several celebrations, including my son's twenty-third birthday, along with three other friends who have birthdays on this date, March 21, 1985 — our shared date.

As I view the current television programs and scan the neighborhoods, I see those who are far more physically challenged than I am. I salute them.

I am not a person who enjoys reliving personal trauma. I do not enjoy the feelings that it revives: pain, struggle, loss of freedom, loss of control, loss of wholeness, helplessness. Yet, because of my dream of becoming a Doctor of Psychology, it was necessary to relive my past pain, putting it on paper for examination, dissection, and criticism. As I see it, my personal reward will be further healing, through exploring the havoc that happened.

Lately, I have thought, perhaps this havoc has been my intermission from my mission; for I had dreamed of attaining my doctorate for years, and was scholastically prepared. My purpose became heightened: my major objective is to guide others who have had either a personal challenge that requires overcoming; or those who face similar challenges that demand the needed ingredients for growth and change. I consider myself a "guideologist" (my invented neologism).

It is not easy to overcome something, or to change, or yet, to find a recipe for success. Hidden somewhere in my studies, the following adages manifested themselves: "If a person wants to change, he or she will" or "They are doing the best they can; otherwise they would be doing something different." But my own double-A formula made exceptional sense: attitude and action helped me change from victim to victor manifesting post-stroke hope. I hope my story of surviving a stroke inspires those who are beginning a similar painful journey. I wish their family members who support and share the burden, and those in the helping healing professions who would like a personal perspective about people whose life has been so suddenly and painfully thrown off course, to understand that this destruction is far greater than can be studied.

It is more than a physical journey to overcome the setbacks of my stroke, which continues to be manifested in the paralysis and uselessness of my left hand. It's a journey of finding my wholeness — wholeness of being. I can also say, it is like a prolonged, convoluted, circuitous detour toward finding my independence, as a person in this culture, at this time of my life.

Ultimately, it became my reason for being: to find this lost aspect of myself. Never have I been an independent person, of independent means and mind. This journey deserves a brief history.

Chapter 1

HISTORY

childhood

MY LINEAGE IS ROOTED IN ANCESTRY OF GERMAN HERITAGE, ENCOMPASSING my father, nephew of the renowned German theologian, Rudolf Otto, who wrote the still-esteemed book *The Idea of the Holy*, among many other profound, spiritual books. My father, his namesake, the eldest of five siblings, immigrated to the United States from the Canary Islands. His father was a German medical doctor in Tenerife. His mother, my grandmother, was born in Bombay, India, of English parents; her father was once the English ambassador to India. Her brother-in-law was the knighted Sir Harry Champion. Grandmother was poetic, esoteric, and spiritual.

My mother came from hearty midwestern stock, who pioneered their way west, settling eventually in Anaheim, at a time when the county of Orange, California, was burgeoning. Mother, domineering and demanding until the day she died at 88, met my sweet-tempered, imaginative father while on an engineering assignment in the dry desert of Trona, California.

My father was my hero, the light of my young life. He inspired me with creative stories he'd invent as we walked in our Alhambra neighborhood, always following dinner, which was always served with lighted candles and linen napkins. Sometimes I sat on his shoulders, propped up, seeing the world from a different, distant vantage point. He taught me about the stars, nature's secrets, emphasizing through his stories, "One can do anything, if she believes in herself" and "it's okay to dream." At least that's the gist I received from his amazing, original fairy tales. As a toddler, I used to sneak away from home, surprising him on his way home from work. I couldn't wait to be with him.

Once, someone discovered me kneeling, with my ears resting on the railroad tracks, listening, waiting for the Red Car to arrive which returned him from a hiking trip. Mother, aware of my disappearance, frantically sought the advice of a "psychic" neighbor for solving her "lost child mystery." I called this dear neighbor "Auntie Chapman." She told mother where I was, just in time to rescue me from the oncoming train!

Father's reputation in the neighborhood was that he walked "ram rod straight," which stemmed from his early, proper German schooling. When he was proud of me he'd pound his chest vigorously, like proud primates in the wild. I passed this tradition on to my children. Daddy and I went hiking on Sundays (just the two of us), but he began staying home too much of the time.

One day I found him lying in the opposite direction on his yellow bedspread, and I asked him, "Daddy, people don't die until they get gray hair, do they?"

He answered calmly, slowly, with a tear glistening in the corner of his eye, "No, my dear daughter," he said, "that's not true." It was during that conversation that he continued speaking in his soft, German accented voice, saying, "Martha Jane, I want you, as eldest daughter, to take care of Mommy, and Mary — always."

My sister Mary was four years younger than I. I didn't quite understand, at that time, why he said those words. This request sounded odd, so foreign, so strange. And yet, I felt so secure with him. But I later learned and understood what it meant. He suffered from a melanoma on his tanned, athletic back. On the unforgettable date of January 23, 1945 (1/2/3/4/5) — he died. The cancer had spread in four years to his liver. He was 49. I was 8. I learned of his death, brutally.

Our next-door neighbor, Velma, appeared at school holding hands with my sister Mary. We three were to walk home together. This was peculiar, I thought; it had never happened before. As I stepped off the curb on the sidewalk, Velma announced: "When you go home, your daddy won't be there, because he died."

These words felt like a sharp, hot knife, stabbing deep into my chest. I screamed, "Oh no!" I ran as fast as I could. I ran past my home, where I saw Mother standing on the front lawn, still in her brown bathrobe, arms folded across her chest. She looked like a stiff broom. I ran past Mother, entering my dear friend Joan's house, screaming and sobbing: "My daddy died! My daddy died!"

Tenderly, Joan said, "Well, now my father can be your father." As gracious as her offer was, it caused me greater pain. Her father was always in a state of rage.

I was never to be the same after that date. It changed and shaped what I thought, how I felt, for the remainder of my life.

Since this is not a book describing grief, per se, I shall jump to other events acquainting the reader with my past persona.

adolescence

My independent, strong, domineering and demanding mother "pulled the curtain down," as she described it, moved to a snooty, suburban San Marino neighborhood, sharing a house with her mother. We moved there when I was 10. I left my memories and secure Alhambra neighborhood and friends to whom I had attached myself and had grown to love very deeply. I entered a cold, cliquish crowd that caused me abysmal pain and suffering. No one knew. I could not connect with the new students. The popular group called The Red Coats always wore red jackets, so they could easily be recognized by their peers from afar on the playground. I distanced myself behind the chain-linked fence and stared at them, shivering in my loneliness.

During this time I gained an enormous amount of weight, which for a child can be devastating. With buck teeth and white eyelashes, I felt huge, ugly, and isolated, to the extreme of having no friends. Consequently, I'd hide in the girls' lavatory and sit on the cold tile floor, eating my lunch — by myself — every day.

Beginning at the age of five, it was the tradition for me to take piano lessons, which later proved to be important for two reasons. While my sister Mary had her lesson, I'd wander up the street to a market where I sat on the magazine rack's wooden ledge reading comic books. There was an awfully grumpy pharmacist who continuously shouted at me: "You can't sit there and read those comics! You must pay for them, first." I'd hide my head in shame, sit on the curb silently sobbing, wishing I had a friend.

When it was my turn for my piano lesson, sometimes I practiced with another girl, and we'd play two-piano duets. I admired her for her physical beauty. Later, she became Homecoming

Queen of South Pasadena High School — a school I soon would enter, as San Marino didn't have a high school yet.

While sitting alone on the curb, escaping the screaming pharmacist, I imagined how wonderful it would be to be crowned Homecoming Queen. I dreamed I did, which was a childish but fun fantasy. It occupied my time.

One day when Mother was driving Mary and me home from our piano lessons, Mother suddenly twirled her head around, after stopping at a signal, announcing she was going to marry the awful, grumpy pharmacist. I was in shock and severely stunned at this far-out surprise. Quickly, I became angry with rage and disbelief, violently screaming loudly: "You can't do that! He's awful! He's horrid! And I hate him!" I was 15 years old at that time. Apparently, Mother had been flirting with him while I had my piano lesson, but I was unaware. My unaccustomed rage surprised me, even though it solved nothing. Mother strongly followed her announcement by saying, "It's my life, and I'll do what I want." This left me feeling hollow. I swallowed my emptiness and daydreamed even further.

When the San Marino students entered the South Pasadena High School we merged quietly, making new friends in the halls that echoed with their well-established cliques.

I had a secret plan. I decided, since I had few friends, that perhaps by changing my image I could acquire new friends in this new environment. My braces were removed during the summer before I entered; I had learned how to apply makeup and mascara to cover my embarrassing white eyelashes and had lost some of my "baby fat." After the makeover, I felt better about my image when I looked into the mirror, studying a different-looking person who appeared almost glamorous. I changed my name from Martha to Marty. My goal was to become Homecoming Queen —

a dream I still harbored in my heart. Therefore, I advanced my plan by making one friend in each clique, which soon began mushrooming into so many friends I didn't know which one to speak to first upon entering the campus, not wanting to offend anyone.

Soon, I was feeling a powerful surge of self-esteem, something I had never known or felt before. I felt fantastic! Powerful! Profound!

When the nomination of Homecoming Queen was announced, and I found myself walking across the auditorium's stage, my heart pounded with pride. Later, my boyfriend George who was on the voting committee, told me I had won "by a landslide!" I cried with inner triumph, which no one knew. I felt that perhaps my father's innate wisdom had guided me toward success. I had won, on my own, with his help, accomplishing something that I had visualized for many years. I rode in the 1955 Tournament of Roses Parade on South Pasadena's float as "The Bird in the Gilded Cage" — another memory I treasure. No one knew what a happy and proud bird was singing and swinging in the cage — a metaphor that only my inner self can vocalize.

This was a major lesson in my life, a lesson that said: "Whatever you want, you can achieve."

This lesson helped me graduate from Whittier College with straight A's. I needed my own inner motivation to accomplish that new goal, since I allowed my high school political career to rob me of valuable study time; and I needed to make up for this lost time. Fortunately, for my future, I planned my education around Sociology/Psychology/Education.

adult

During a summer break, as a Sociology major, I traveled with the first exchange students entering Russia. It was one of the most valuable inner experiences of my young life. Upon returning home, I was commissioned by a neighborhood newspaper to write articles about my Russian experiences.

After graduating from college, I married a law student, soon to become an attorney, whom I helped put through law school by teaching elementary school. I taught sixth grade juvenile delinquents in an unsafe Los Angeles neighborhood, later transferring to a more prosperous neighborhood when my lawyer spouse changed his daytime job; there, I was challenged by gifted students.

A few years later I had a son, then a daughter, 16 months apart. Subsequently, my spouse became an alcoholic, whose binges left me whimpering and frightened. I was unwilling to live the rest of my life trusting his pattern would change. We divorced. I decided that was his process; I had mine; my future life would be happy, for I thought I was in charge of my destiny.

I became a student of numerology, the arts, a novice writer, eventually marrying my second husband whom I met at a friend's party. It was a romantic encounter, a chemistry that literally connected us "across a crowded room." He was a Hollywood television producer, well known in his arena. The first photograph at the end of this book depicts us before attending an Emmy ceremony. It is significant to insert at this point that today, as I write this, we have celebrated our 25th wedding anniversary. This marriage has been my true gift in life; for we have learned how to become the "blended" family: he with his three children, plus his cat, and I with my two children, and now (at this writing) eleven grandchildren fulfilling our cycle.

During the early years of our married life, in the '70s, I did many things: I worked as a television extra, and part-time Production Assistant on the situation comedy "Sanford and Son"; wrote a book, *Child Inside Me*, which was published by Grosset and Dunlap; developed my arts and crafts business, followed by my videotape/editing hobby, gradually growing a business in that field.

One day during a long hike in our Hollywood Hills area, I listened to my inner voice, a quiet voice that often spoke to me in a clear, distinct manner: "It's now time for you to return to graduate school." With a friend's guidance, I found a perfect, stimulating school, California Family Study Center, in my area that specialized in the study of Marriage/Family/Child Counseling. In addition, as it turned out, two friends, Diane and Judy, were also enrolling. We three bespectacled older women, aged 47, felt the excitement of education in the highest sense. It was a new adventure. I was euphoric!

I marveled at the joy I felt at this stimulating challenge, and excelled there. I even raised my hand to speak out loud in front of my peers for the first time in my life! What had happened to the shy, timid, withdrawn little person I once was? Was this what mature people felt? I didn't know. Furthermore, it didn't matter; I kept on going. I stopped smoking, I ate healthy food, eliminating all red meats. My hikes in the hills grew longer. I enjoyed the new beauty of nature, especially when huffing and puffing up the steep hills that surrounded our home. I felt alive, almost high, and wanting more exercise. Therefore, my heart also pounded to Jane Fonda's heavy-duty workout video in my home. I huffed and puffed like the little engine that could.

However, I neglected to stop long enough to question the peculiar blackness that would fall over my right eye, like a curtain, as well as the early-morning numbness in my right hand. This usually happened after exercise, but always diminished within a few minutes. Why should I bother to acknowledge these silly symptoms? I felt fantastic. I felt better than ever.

While preparing to attend a much anticipated weekend workshop at my school, I suddenly felt seriously ill. Unfortunately, our family doctor had recently died. Therefore, wanting to be well for the workshop, I instructed my husband to take me to the hospital emergency room. He agreed.

Chapter 2

ALARMING NEWS

the doctor's visit

THE ATTENDING PHYSICIAN AT THE EMERGENCY HOSPITAL EXAMINED ME, VERIFYING the fact that I, indeed, had the Philippine Flu, instructing me to go home, "Drink lots of fluids, and get plenty of bed rest. . . ." — the usual home remedy prescription. However, his last comment was, "If you're not well by Tuesday, I suggest you see a doctor." I explained that our family doctor had died. He gave me a sheet with a list of doctors in our area. While examining this long list, I thought to myself, I'm not going to see a strange doctor I know nothing about. As if guided by an invisible force, my eyes focused on a familiar name — Dr. King — a doctor my husband's children had used in the past. Relieved, I went home and waited to see how I'd feel by the following Tuesday.

When the following Tuesday came, I felt better, but my inner voice spoke to me again, this time firmly saying, "Go to the doctor." Trusting this voice, I made an appointment with Dr. King.

Dr. King officially verified that I had the Philippine Flu, and wrote a prescription. While I was holding this piece of paper, he removed his stethoscope and began to position it onto the right side of my neck, holding it for what seemed like a very long time. I was puzzled as to why he held it there for so long and asked him what he was doing. I watched his face grow ashen as he plopped down onto the small stool on rollers. Again I repeated, "What's going on?"

He said matter-of-factly, "You have absolutely no pulse in the right side of your body."

"My God! What does that mean?" I asked, feeling rather unsteady.

"You may have a blockage," he answered.

Not wanting to panic, I explained that, "After exercise, my right eye becomes black, as if a curtain fell over it, and in the morning my right hand is sometimes numb."

His voice sounded calm, but controlled. "Hmmm, that sounds like a classic case of Takayasus Disease," he added.

"Taki *what*?" I heard myself trying to copy his foreign word.

"Takayasus Disease," he repeated. "It was discovered by a Japanese doctor, whose last name, Takayasus, was used to distinguish it. It is a rare disease that is being discovered in more and more American women your age," he added, continuing now with a faster-paced voice. He described that this rare disease is an inflammation in the arteries and veins that has a residual effect of forming scar tissue on the inside of the artery, thus creating a blockage that affects the blood flow.

While he was offering this explanation, I found my mind wandering, not completely listening to his words. They all seemed to run together. I felt stunned and weak, only partially hearing these alarming sentences. "What does this mean?" I managed to mutter.

"This means you will need to have an examination by a vascular surgeon, probably an angiogram to determine the extent of the blockage. And then we'll go from there." He finalized my examination by telling me he was going on a two-week vacation, and gave me his vascular surgeon colleague's name and number, Dr. Sethi. I was instructed to contact him while he was gone. As I exited his office, I felt shaky and confused and decided to phone my husband at work. I explained the alarming news, not wanting to seem upset or panicked, although needing his comfort and support. He gave me just what I wanted, saying, "We'll do what needs to be done." I hung up feeling soothed, but still shaky.

During the two weeks while Dr. King was on vacation, I saw Dr. Sethi, a Pakistani doctor, well accepted in his profession. He seemed equally concerned, and had me schedule an angiogram immediately.

the angiogram

The night before this procedure, I was lying in the hospital bed reading an exciting text from my school that read like a novel. It was Carl Whitaker's *The Family Crucible*. It kept my interest, diverting my anxiety. Suddenly there was a phone call from my stepson, Shaun. He had never called me before. I put the book down and listened to his comforting words. They made me feel good. During this rare conversation, I told him I couldn't believe I was having this experience. I said that maybe if it were Dad, I could understand, but not me. Shaun very wisely said, "Perhaps you're having it for Dad."

After hanging up the phone, I picked up the book to continue reading. In the very next sentence the words I read said exactly the same as those Shaun had said, the essence of which were: "When two people are close, one person sometimes unconsciously has things happen to him for the other person, instead of the other person having it." I felt the power of synchronicity speaking to me — again.

The angiogram procedure was an uncomfortable experience. As I lay on the cold table, I looked at the white ceiling, counting the squares, feeling frightened, not believing I was really having this done; not believing something that drastic was wrong. While the dye was flowing through my veins, I felt as though the top of my head was going to explode. I cried out, "Stop! Stop! Please, stop!"

The technician said, "I'm so sorry, but we need to do it again."

Consequently, again the top of my head felt as though it was going to explode. I closed my eyes, and prayed.

the doctor's report

The results of the angiogram were not good. The test revealed that my right carotid artery had a 94% blockage — a blockage that was severe and seriously alarming. This sudden news left me feeling numb, dazed, incoherent. I didn't think this kind of thing could happen to me. Other people, yes; but not me. I was only 48, living a happy, and what I had thought was a healthy, life.

Chapter 3

BYPASS
SURGERY SCURRY

the night before

IT WAS THE EVE OF MY BYPASS SURGERY. I FELT NOTHING SPECIAL, EXCEPT I wished the surgery would be over. I had phoned Dr. Sethi at some point before the surgery date asking him what was going to happen. I must have caught him at a difficult time for he answered me with, "Don't rush my study. I must examine it carefully, for your case is very tricky, very complicated."

I impatiently waited for my husband, Norm, to arrive in my hospital room. Dr. Sethi had arrived earlier than expected, furrowed his brow below his colorful turban, and began to explain the presurgery and operation details. I stopped his monologue in midword; I didn't want him repeating the information twice. When Norm arrived, we listened to the doctor's words, barely hearing him state that strokes could happen as a result of this kind of procedure. We nodded, sighing.

Dr. Sethi also explained that he would insert a Dacron mesh synthetic artery above my aorta, bypassing the blocked artery, crisscrossing over the carotid artery. He explained he would also saw open my sternum, pulling it apart, to form a cave they would work in, leaving a zipper-like scar. I figured this completed my bikini wearing days, even though I reluctantly knew the end had terminated somewhat earlier. Only Playboy Bunny, supermodel older persons wear bikinis. This was not I. However, I didn't imagine not wearing a low-cut blouse anymore (or playing the flute, which I taught myself).

Nevertheless, the procedure sounded complicated. Dr. Sethi and Norm shook hands, vowing they'd meet following surgery. I asked Norm to put my wedding ring onto my finger, so I'd know he was there after the surgery. He said he would, and slid it into his pocket, kissed me, and turned to leave the room. Before he left, we gave each other our favorite three hand-squeezes ritual which says "I love you." Then as he walked out the door, I blew him a silent kiss, gave a two-handed wave from my bed, with both thumbs up, just like the astronauts do before their takeoff.

After he left, I felt anxiety mounting, so I scurried into the bathroom where I cleansed my face and put on mascara. I didn't want anyone to see my white eyelashes — a foolish carryover from my bland past. I didn't fool the specialists the next day, however. They asked me to remove it, before instructing me to put on the green surgical cap. My new life was about to begin, I pondered.

Chapter 4

LIFE CHANGES IN AN INSTANT

intensive care unit

VAGUELY, I RECALL SQUINTING AT THE HUGE, ROUND, WHITE LIGHTS, PROTRUDING like flying saucers, perched somewhere in the ceiling . . . and seeing an orange table beneath my hospital gown . . . then feeling its vinyl-like coldness. The next thing I recall in my foggy, dreamlike state was the amplified voice of Dr. Sethi saying, "Oh my God, she's had a stroke. Move your foot, Martha, move your foot."

Is it over? I thought. I tried to move my foot. Where was my foot? Where was Norm, I wondered. He was not speaking to me. I could not feel my wedding band on my finger. I had asked him earlier to place it on my finger after surgery was done so I'd know he was there; but I learned later he still had it in his pocket. My fingers were too swollen for any rings. I could not feel my finger. "Did someone mention stroke? I don't know what a stroke is."

I tried to talk, but my words sounded garbled, like a lost bird, warbling in the wrong nest. I tried to say, "When my girlfriend Diane's mother had a stroke, they opened up her brain and drained the blood out. Can this be done for me?"

I heard Dr. Sethi say, "Perhaps." His voice sounded strange. It echoed louder than normal, appearing distorted. I heard him speak on my right side.

a scene from a horror movie

That's all I remember in this foggy haze. Later, I learned Norm was standing on my left side. I couldn't see him due to my newly acquired "left-side neglect" caused from the brain injury. People who have had a right-hemisphere stroke may experience one-sided neglect, which may cause them to "forget" or "ignore" objects or people on their left side.

Norm had given me our three "I love you" hand-squeezes; I couldn't feel them. Dr. Sethi was in a closed-off booth in the Intensive Care Unit behind a window observing my postoperative behavior. I was in ICU coming out of the anesthetic.

My family told me that my son, Randy, came and fed me. It was his 23rd birthday — a birthday he will always remember. My daughter, Jennifer, came with her friend, Karen. She told me they walked around the beds three times and couldn't find me. I looked horrid, different, grotesque. This was not her mother. My swollen face, scrunched to the right; my eyes locked to the right; my left hand in a fetal position, resting limply, somewhere. "It was worse than a horror movie," Jennifer later remarked.

At first, I suffered from aphasia, which is the loss or reduction of the ability to speak, read, write, or understand, due to dysfunction of brain centers.

I dimly recall a harsh voice making me cough. "Cough hard," it shouted. "Cough again." "Again!" These commands and tone of voice sounded like a drill sergeant. It was the respiratory therapist who cried out these brutal instructions so my lungs wouldn't collect fluid. I couldn't cough. My chest hurt. It hurt from deep within. I had to breathe rapidly into a tube, which also hurt from deep inside.

I did not know then, but on that day — March 21, 1985 — my life changed in an instant. It is surmised that, during the bypass surgery, a blood clot became lodged in the new mesh artery. When the metal clamp was unlocked, the new blood flow dislodged the clot, projecting it like a rocket to the brain, directly resulting in a stroke in the right hemisphere's abstract perceptual area. It was about 45 minutes after surgery. I almost made it.

my stroke education begins

According to the National Stroke Association, stroke is defined as a "brain attack."

I learned the brain is divided into four primary parts: the right hemisphere (or half), the left hemisphere (or half), the cerebellum and the brain stem. (Please refer to the Appendix for a detailed description of various types of strokes and their specific results.)

I was ultimately diagnosed as having had an ischemic stroke in the right hemisphere, which in simple terms means that vital blood flow in my brain was cut off or reduced by a blood clot and injured part of the right side of my brain.

Chapter 5

MARGARET AND SUSAN

awareness of paralysis

IT WAS DARK WHEN I CONSCIOUSLY DETERMINED I WAS IN A BED. I KNEW IT WAS in the hospital, yet I couldn't understand why I couldn't move my left side. It felt peculiar. I felt my left side, but didn't feel it because there was no feeling in it. In the chaos of my mind, I heard sounds in the room. It sounded like a rustling noise. My hearing seemed to be hyperalert — unusual for blabbermouth Marty.

A soft light outside the heavy door ushered in a crack of light through the hinges. I felt a presence beside me. My eyes finally focused on a figure in white. I sensed the slight movement of my bed, like a tremor before a major earthquake. The covers on my bed began to shift. I was not doing the moving. A soft, sweet voice whispered in the dark. "Hi, Martha. I'm Margaret, your night nurse."

I felt comforted hearing her voice, knowing I was not alone in the darkness. Likewise, I tried to respond by answering her back, but the words caught in my throat; also, I had trouble finding the right words to say. I struggled for a while, until Margaret spoke again, touching my right arm while adjusting my covers. Her touch was light, her voice as gentle as a trade wind. "Do you wonder," she whispered softly, "why you can't move your left side and can't speak the words you want to say?" she asked in this hushed, little girl voice.

At least someone understands me, even in this whispered darkness, I thought. "Yes. Yes," I stammered, struggling.

"You've had a stroke," she whispered again, ever so lightly. "That's the reason you can't move your left side, or have such trouble talking."

"Will I be better by tomorrow?" I figured I'd ask her, just in case she was Florence Nightingale, or a miracle worker.

I don't remember her reply; but her softness, her gentle spirit was as soothing as a warm bath, and made me feel better, whether tomorrow came or not.

my roommate

The brightness of tomorrow seemed wicked. Its harshness harnessed a gloom that left me hovering in my hospital bed: bruised, confused, still groggy from the surgery aftereffects. It was morning when I heard a cheerful female voice that was in the bed next to the window. "Hi," she said.

Surprised, and more confused, I looked over to my right, and in my misty mind, said: "Hi, Diane."

It was not Diane, but Susan, my hospital roommate. She was there, I felt, as a blessing, my personal gift. As time mellowed my pain, we became best friends, supporting each other's every move. Her story, however, was sad.

Susan was admitted into Northridge Hospital, January 11,

1985, after a car accident. The police were in pursuit of a drunk in a pickup truck. The truck hit her car directly, resulting in a collision. Instantly, she became a paraplegic, her entire life put on hold. She was, and still is, unable to use her legs, due to her spinal cord injury. She left her home one night to return a video; in doing this, her life drastically changed, forever.

Susan and I shared all our hospital drama together: from good and bad hospital food, to good and bad TV programs. We learned each other's history, met each other's friends, family, and doctors. We enjoyed each other's flowers, brought by supporters. We conferred on our medications, gossiped about the nurses, complained about the noise, the hospital system: sharing secrets, giggling, like silly little girls.

the michael jackson glove; and i'm "doing it"

Susan's watch alarm beeped on the hour, usually waking us up in the middle of the night at the same time. We'd cry, talk in our sleep, or discuss some weird dream in the darkness. Upon awaking in the morning, we interpreted each other's dreams. Also, she liked coffee; I liked herb tea. When I'd lose my glasses, she'd remind me to, "Look on your left side," and there they'd be. My left-side neglect caused this omission. The doctors put a glove on my left hand, preventing it from becoming too spastic. Susan and I called it my "Michael Jackson Glove."

When Susan thought she had moved her toes slightly, once, I bought her a pink sweatshirt that said across the front in white letters, "I'm doing it." Someone took a snapshot of us to remember this event. We both would leave on our daily missions to therapy (rehab), in our wheelchairs, except Susan was better at maneuvering hers.

Chapter 6

"HUMPTY DUMPTY," "STROKE LADY" AND "CLAW"

"wheelchairing"

THE DOCTORS STARTED ME IN REHABILITATION THERAPY IMMEDIATELY. According to American Heart/Stroke Association literature, the quicker the rehab program starts, the faster the recovery. In fact, someone pointed out to me that the most promising recovery is done within the first six months. I was told, "Whatever recovery is achieved during the first year will probably be the only recovery achieved, for a while."[3]

I dispute this theory, as this speculation only documented

---

[3] See Meerwaldt in the Bibliography.

hearsay at that time; my recovery shows otherwise. I'm still making progress after 10 years!

However, to get to the rehabilitation station, I needed to "drive" myself. This meant maneuvering in a wheelchair. I cannot describe the torture I endured, trying to make it go around corners, in and out of crowded elevators — all with one hand.

Often, I felt like giving up. It was a fight to find a place in the packed elevators, seemingly choked with other wheelchairs, especially before the doors closed. They closed fast. To reach for the elevator button was a challenge. The elevator buttons needed designs with wheelchair ease in mind.

discouragement and depression

When I finally arrived at the rehabilitation area, many times I felt drained of any energy.[4] The physical therapists would transfer my body from wheelchair to table, which at first was only about a foot off the ground. The tables were orange vinyl, similar to the surgery table I described earlier, except lower. Some of the higher tables had parallel bars attached, which I learned to use eventually.

Rehabilitation therapy was a new, unwanted, yet needed experience. Some experts have expressed grave doubts about these therapeutic services, believing that little evidence exists to support their success.[5]

My first encounter with this rehabilitation therapy consisted of sitting on the edge of the one-foot table. I felt as though I was almost sitting on the floor. However, when I sat down I'd roll over

---

[4] See Newman in the Bibliography.
[5] See Hachinski in the Bibliography.

to one side, usually my right, unable to keep my balance. Norm lovingly called me Humpty-Dumpty. I couldn't sit up by myself.

My speaking also sounded slurred to me, as I'd hear a staccato voice trying to communicate to others. Likewise, I'd have difficulty getting the words out, and finding the right words to use.[6]

This presentation seemed to continue day after day, endlessly. I'd work until I'd cry in utter despair; yet, the therapists made me go beyond this point of protest. Often I felt discouraged, as I hated the torture of this attempt to regain my old physical image. I felt angry. I thought there was no proof, no evidence, that my body would ever respond, except for the sixth-month report, as told to me by someone.

Depression in stroke patients is expected and common. The research literature is replete with evidence documenting depression's disastrous disability in stroke patients. Although these findings could result in an entire written document, suffice it to say that the short-term and long-term consequences of depression symptoms range from mild to severe, and deserves detailed attention for those interested.[7]

The relative frequency of major and minor depressive syndromes among patients with post-stroke depression has varied among studies.

encouragement

I had much encouragement from Dr. Sethi, who visited me daily on his rounds. Acting like a coach, he would say, "You can do

---

[6] See Messner and Messner, and Ross in the Bibliography.
[7] See Messner and Messner, Newman, and Robinson, et al. in the Bibliography.

it. You will do it. And you're doing it." My children and husband added their encouragement too. Son Randy quipped, "Mom, remember: no pain, no gain." Daughter Jennifer laughingly called me "Stroke Lady," which at the time I learned to love. Later she'd tease me by calling me, "Mother Martyr," which seemed also appropriate.

Norm and I called my stroke hand "Claw" — which remains in our vocabulary today. Norm tells me that Claw reminded him of the actor, Peter Sellers, in the movie, "Dr. Strange Love," when the black-gloved hand suddenly flew up spontaneously, giving the salute, "Heil Hitler," with Peter Sellers trying to grab it with the opposite hand, bringing it under control. It's certainly true — Claw had, and continues to have, its own personality: getting caught in jackets, making it difficult for even another person to disengage it. Sometimes, it seems like a three-handed game. As the hospital rehabilitation plan continued, there were other activities to endure, further challenges to meet . . . all at once . . . all in time.

It is imperative to insert at this juncture the value of social support for stroke patients, hinted above, as well as documented in the forthcoming sections.

As with the excessive amount of material on depression, so it is with the issue of social support. Despite findings that indicate the beneficial effects of social support, recent evidence suggests that some interactions with others have deleterious effects on the victims of life crisis.

The sudden onset of stroke often represents a threat to the adaptive and coping abilities of patients. The nature and severity of cognitive/intellectual, affective, and sensorimotor functioning often render stroke patients dependent and elicit attempts to help from family and friends. In addition to enhancing the ability of older people to cope with physical decline, assistance from social network members may also hamper these efforts (for example, concerns by others for patients' health, overprotectiveness, and preferential treatment of patients experiencing heart disease and a variety of other chronic illnesses.

Furthermore, it is believed that negative and positive interactions demonstrated greater improvement in cognitive functioning after discharge from the hospital. It is possible that encouragement and reinforcement perceived by these patients stimulated mental activity and resulted in improved orientation.

My social support team encouraged me to go beyond my obvious limits; thus, my work was just beginning.

Chapter 7

OTHER ACTIVITIES, FURTHER CHALLENGES

compulsions

DIRECTLY AFTER THE STROKE, MY MIND BEGAN TO CHANGE IN TERMS OF MY thinking process. I was keenly aware of this. As an example, my thought patterns operated like a filing system. I never experienced this organizational-likeness thinking before. However, I considered myself organized; even if organized in a disorganized fashion. In the hospital, I needed to have things right at my arm's reach — the right hand reach. Things had to be in a certain place, usually driving everyone crazy. If certain items like my water glass or tissue box were not within this direct reach radius, I would experience anxiety. My hypothesis is that my left brain began compensating immediately. This structure need still applies today.

Some of my research confirmed that "obsessive and compulsive behaviors including counting objects and stereotyped motor behavior have been observed."[8]

tantrums

My emotions were raw. I'd cry over the silliest things, as well as over the most profound tragedies. The Iran hostage crisis, happening at that time, had me sobbing. Unconsciously, and metaphorically, I felt like a hostage in my own body and mind.

This impulsiveness continued after I returned home. Often I would have a tantrum, which was not like the "old Marti." Once I thought I lost a pair of Ice scissors, a professional brand of well-honed barber scissors. I looked everywhere, yet didn't really need them for any particular reason. This loss compulsively caused me immediately to persuade my father-in-law to drive me to the beauty supply house to buy another pair, for $25.00. It was ridiculous, in retrospect, but appeared significant at the time. Perhaps symbolically, I wanted to find my cutoff lost self, or couldn't tolerate my cutoff lost self, wishing to replace it with a sense of wholeness.

ulcers

While in the hospital I also acquired a magnified case of ulcers, which prevented me from eating. The pain was severe, and familiar. I had had a less severe case a few years earlier, and therefore, was unpleasantly accustomed to this pain. A gastroenterologist examined my stomach through an endoscopy, resulting in an

---

[8] See Crosile, et al. in the Bibliography.

expressive verbal comment at what he saw : "Oh my God, no wonder!"

The ulcers were covering my entire stomach lining. Yes, there was no wonder why I had such stomach pains. No wonder I was unable to eat. No wonder I was wasting away. The proper medication corrected this condition, with the doctor informing me this was not unusual in my stroke circumstances. "It happens frequently," he said, although I was unable to locate evidence to support this hypothesis.

After returning to my hospital room from this endoscopy procedure, I found a big, colorful balloon awaiting me at the foot of my bed. Apparently, Bill, Norm's boat partner and friend, came for a visit, found me gone and left his welcome gift floating toward the ceiling. This was a much-needed lift, symbolically as well. Another charming present — a surprise scent — was on my pillow, while I was sleeping: a small, dainty, fragrant sachet nosegay, delivered by an anonymous hospital volunteer. Whomever that anonymous person was had no idea how happy that made me feel.

There were low times when these simple treats, unadorned pleasures and sweet treasures comforted a very lonely and sad heart. The importance of these actions was confirmed in my research when I discovered that "following stroke, perception of social support from key relationships may mediate the emotional response to this life crisis."[9]

a neurologist's prediction

A neurologist gave me a gloomy prediction, after explaining

---

[9] See Morris, Robinson, et al. in the Bibliography.

the area of my brain that had been injured. He drew a comprehensive diagram and took the time to illustrate the facts of my injury in detail. Consequently, this satisfied my curiosity and my desire for knowledge; but he destroyed any brave spirit that was brewing below the bleak surface. He walked from my hospital bed, strolled down the corridor, turning his head back in my direction and saying almost as an aside: "You may never get the use of your left-hand fingers back."

Knowing how much past satisfaction I had received from writing and typing, I became ripe with anger. I shot up in bed, like a spring, at a straight right-angled sitting position, shouting as he continued walking down the hall: "You'll see! I'll show you! I'll show you!"

He had earlier told me I might never be able to drive a car again, which left me in a quiet mood for quite some time.

more rehabilitation

I took speech therapy, occupational and physical therapy. The speech therapist had me working on a computer, telling me it would help heal my brain. I played simple games which occupied my time. The most enjoyment I had was in occupational therapy. I used a typewriter with one hand. It was a manual clunker, but I didn't mind. I could express myself by writing letters, describing my imprisonment. I was able to do this when I finished with their puzzles, which I disliked. I couldn't figure them out. They represented my perception deficits, which I didn't understand at that time, and therefore left me thinking that I must be stupid.[10]

---

[10] See Thompson, et al. in the Bibliography.

During this phase, I took a battery of tests, including the Wechsler Intelligence Scale and Luria-Nebraska Neuropsychological battery. They became highly anxiety provoking. During the perception part, I felt even more uptight, more stupid, especially when confronted with the "Block Designs." When it came to the mathematics section, I raised my hand in total defiance. I told the patient examiner that I'd never been proficient in math, questioning him as to why I should be now, and rested my head on the table, like a sullen teenager, crying. I must have scored very low in my Intelligence Quotient score.

At that time, I gave up, feeling highly unintelligent for the first time, as though I was from some foreign planet. It was a low point. When he quizzed me on plot and story detail, I totally failed. As this had been my past video/movie profession, I was certain my life was over. This devastated my being, causing any hope for inner peace to plummet.

Brain studies have demonstrated that "the predominant feature of confusion was an executive incoherence. Right-hemisphere patients tended to have great difficulty developing, pursuing and modifying a course of action in mental arithmetic problems and in construction tasks."[11] Research also suggests that "spatial ability tests (such as the Block Design test) can be solved by either a verbal-analytic ('left' hemisphere) strategy or a spatial-holistic ('right' hemisphere) strategy." This confusion has been referred to as "Constructional Apraxia, the inability to produce designs in two or three dimensions, by copying, drawing or construction upon command or spontaneously."[12]

---

[11] See Calvanio, et al. in the Bibliography.
[12] See Bjorneby and Reinvang in the Bibliography.

dressing

Equally important to my health and survival, but causing great embarrassment, was trying to teach myself to dress. I could not even understand how to put on my underpants. Imagine, I thought, after 48 years, I can't even figure out how to put on a pair of panties. Now I know how children or the elderly must feel, with their faculties not developed or having declined.

It was not only my perception that seemed injured, but my spirit, my pride felt wounded as well. The underpants looked strange, unfamiliar. I couldn't figure out which was front and which was back. In addition, to put on underwear with one hand was impossible.

The occupational therapist was patient and understanding, walking me through this gruesome nightmare, over and over, day after day. I only wore different colored sweatpants and matching tennies and socks — which Norm chose, by himself. The tennis shoes had to be with Velcro fasteners, for tying shoelaces with one hand was impossible. Try it!

It wasn't until I returned home that my dear Norm taught me an easy way to put my top on, which helped ease my frustration. He showed me by laying the shirt on the bed, with the label up, facing me, saying, "Pretend we are dancing. See, the label goes up," he'd emphasize. To this day, I use his technique.

I am able to understand today that I experienced "dressing apraxia": confusion about the orientation of clothing. One of my research sources reported that "copying ability correlates with dressing skills, and with final dressing performance."[13] Another

---

[13] See Bell, et al. in the Bibliography.

source taught me that "kinetic apraxia in the form of loss of fine movements in the non-affected hand predicts a poorer outcome in ADL (activities of daily living) skills."[14]

This is valuable information for me today, since I still struggle with my dressing performance, and often find a lost left shoe somewhere behind my path as I cannot feel if it is on or off my paralyzed foot. Lack of self-confidence in dressing affects self-esteem. Several of my research sources focused on "dressing performance" and the lack of self-confidence in stroke patients. Further research is required to investigate the strategies used to overcome dressing problems, so that patients need not undergo lengthy trial and error procedures.

eating

I also learned how to eat and cut my food with a curved knife that adjusted for one-hand use. Feeding myself was to become a further challenge. Even removing the plastic wrap from the food, with one hand, was a terrible task. But, in time, the loving therapists and nurses educated and retrained me with their proficient professionalism. Their teachings were important lessons for my future survival.

My research uncovered a case study[15] that offers a cognitive prosthesis for self-feeding that I find particularly helpful. It's a hard plastic circular plate with a raised edge around the perimeter and sectioned off in the interior into three sections that can be rotated on a platform similar to a lazy Susan. I find this helpful because I

---

[14] See Diller, et al. in the Bibliography.
[15] See Calvanio, et al. in the Bibliography.

only ate food on the right side of my plate, ignoring the left side due to my left-side neglect. Thus, the lazy Susan device could rotate my eating woes away, leaving me to concentrate consciously on the food on my left side.

bathing

Bathing was also a new challenge. I recall my first bathing experience on my first day in my new hospital bed after ICU. I awoke to a large, obese Black nurse who told me it was bath time. The moment I saw her, her demeanor caused me to feel that I wanted her to hug me. I told her I needed her to hug me. She looked at me with a strange, quizzical facial expression, as if thinking, "You want me to do what?" But she hugged me anyway, and I felt as though I were held in the luxurious arms of a soft pillow. It felt so comforting. I wept with emotion, wishing all my tears and fears would absorb into this softness.

Following her huge hug, she wheeled me into a large room — the bathing room — with tile on the walls and floor. I sat in my wheelchair as she showered, soaped, scrubbed, and rinsed me from head to feet. It was just like washing a car. I had never felt so clean.

I needed to feel this "squeaky clean" feeling, for going to the toilet was sometimes awkward and often embarrassing. Occasionally, I didn't quite make it in time. Summoning the nurses for this task meant waiting . . . waiting while they answered my call, and waiting for them to transfer me from wheelchair to toilet or from bed to bedpan. Once, in the evening, a friend brought me a gift in a lovely, gold gift box. I inadvertently left the empty box on my hospital table during the night. In the morning I realized that in my nighttime confusion I had left my bedpan "gift" in the empty box, grabbing it, by an accident, thinking it was a bedpan! This caused quite a commotion with the nurses. They brought their friends in to view this strange gift. "All it needed," one nurse said, "was a ribbon on top!"

When the relatives of stroke patients are asked about the problems they encounter with the patients, they consistently mention lifting, incontinence and bathing.

antidepressants

At some point during Dr. King's rounds, he queried me, asking if I felt depressed. I thought for a moment. I didn't feel depressed; for when I learned that I'd had a stroke, I said to myself, "Well, I've had a stroke; can I do anything about it? Can I change it?" I said "No," and slithered into a silent acceptance.

But his question triggered a response that surprised me. I responded by saying "Yes," because I'd heard that antidepressant medication helps one to sleep better, and my sleep habits were poor. He prescribed the antidepressant, Amitriptyline. I slept better, but had no idea of the aftereffects when I tried to get off it much later, at home (described in a later section).[16]

other therapies

A favorable adjunct to my therapies was biofeedback.[17] This technique helped me relax, and carried over in my home program. The most valued therapy, the high point of my day, was when

---

[16] See Beckson and Cummings in the Bibliography.

[17] In Calvanio, et al., the treatment benefits in bio-feedback and other behavioral modification methods are discussed in length.

Norm regularly visited me after work. He would help feed me, reminding me I had packed food in the left side of my mouth. He brushed my teeth and wiped my mouth. He helped me practice going to the toilet. He'd read me stories, bring me surprises that helped me smile — my crooked smile. His visits were a pleasant interlude, like a soothing symphony or a retreat, when he was with me.

He was a true treat. His visits were a reminder of home. I'd hear myself sing "The Homesick Blues," when he'd leave, especially toward the end of my hospital stay. On the weekends he'd push me in my wheelchair to the hospital's upper-level solarium or outside patio. Here we would bask in the sun. I'd hear the birds that I longed to hear and missed so much.

This was part of institutional living that finally got to me, becoming my best, and worst, enemy like a dark phantom, or a fun fantasy. The outdoors was my natural, real therapy — a true sanctuary from the encompassing, suffocating reality. I felt the healing process flow through my veins when confronted with sunshine, birds, fresh air, spells of laughter, and Norm. He caused my heart to flutter and my soul to sing. He loaned me his left hand, which became mine. I prayed I would make him smile, a smile that I loved so much, a smile that in itself was a gift — a gift as healing as sunshine. I borrowed it frequently.

Chapter 8

CHEERS, TEARS, HOORAYS AND GOOD-BYES

friends

DESPITE MY DEFECTS, FRIENDS WOULD APPEAR, ALTHOUGH I BARELY SAW THEM. At first, my eyes were locked securely over to my right side.[18] Visitors were encouraged to stand on my left side; so I would train my eyes to focus there. I learned to listen attentively, sometimes hearing on a deeper level, to meanings of comments that I had not registered before. It was unusual. It was fun.

When my friend Phyllis visited me she became so disturbed when she saw me, she excused herself and went to the outside hallway and cried in private. While outside recovering from her initial shock, I

---

[18] Norm said later that he felt horrified. "My God," he wailed," this beautiful woman will kill herself if she sees her eyes like this." Except today he adds, "But I would have loved you anyway." He was an obviously troubled man in love.

heard her chastise a nurse, unfairly, for some unfounded reason. Visibly shaken, she used anyone as a scapegoat for her own despair.

Other dear friends came: Mina, my neighborhood barber, Jean, and Janet, and the Shatz, appeared, offering their smiles, their sunshine, their support. My former Dutch boyfriend Harry, whom I met as a sociology exchange student in 1958, phoned me from Holland, offering cheer. I felt elated, hearing from him (my untread path in life). Family members also showed their continual support, visiting often.

Once while in rehab, I had a surprise visit from Norm's #1 stage property person, Lou Gomovitz, fondly referred to as "Gommie," who worked on his show. He was formerly the director for the puppet show, "Kukla, Fran, and Ollie." Kukla's face was modeled after his. I felt touched by Gommie's interest, sensitivity, and concern, for I didn't know him very well. Friends, family, and their support were like a strong brace that stabilized my floundering, easing the new reality.

There was one fair-weather friend whom I had helped move out from Iowa, who lived in our home for six months. She disappeared. I never heard from her again, despite my numerous phone calls and pleas for her help. Perhaps she saw herself in me, unable to face the truth of her own mortality. Nevertheless, from her I learned about friends — who really were friends and who were not.

My research supported these observations. While supportive interactions with friends can have a positive impact on functioning, unfortunately, decline in functioning results in estrangement from friends.[19]

Another time, a group of Norm's coworkers came. We all met and partied in the lounge on the first floor. I in my wheelchair; they

---

[19] See Norris, et al. in the Bibliography.

seated in the soft designer chairs and couches. We talked, laughed. I felt my face stretch as I smiled. That was a good feeling. The colors in this lobby were my favorite — turquoise and raspberry — causing a comforting, friendly inner feeling, adding new pleasure to this rare merriment.

However, sometimes when my old friends, Diane and Judy, would attempt to visit me, I would not allow them to enter my room, as I was drooling. It was an excuse, because they represented my past graduate school days, when I had felt alive, healthy, and fully functioning. I knew this drooling had an effect on my ego; I felt it was disgusting, not realizing it is common with stroke victims. My vanity was disgusting. I felt embarrassed.

On other visits when loneliness had overcome my ego, Diane and Judy observed, without comment, the tissue-in-the-right-hand cover-up trick. This cover-up fooled no one. Eventually, I learned to accept myself, drooling or not drooling.

Diane gave me a card that read, "When one door closes, another opens." It was impossible to integrate this wisdom at that time. I just wanted to feel normal.

eyes unlocking

One special day, Norm entered through my hospital room door, and stood there for an instant, greeting me with his smile. And, like magic, I felt my eyes pull from the right to the left, following him, focusing on him at the door when he entered. I studied his smile. It felt like having my eyes crossed for a long time, and suddenly strain, pulling them to adjust properly where they belong.

You should have heard Norm's reaction, his exclamation, seen his extended smile. He screamed, "Hooray, hooray, hooray!" The nurses, and it seemed as though everyone else, came to my room to learn what the excitement was. When I moved my eyes again, I saw Norm's eyes, filled with tears. Everyone else's did likewise, and there was a loud series of tearful cheers. It was like the good feeling associated with having a straight shot of green lights when in a hurry driving home.

I didn't realize how far I had come. In the midst of this celebration, I didn't realize the importance of loving friends; an absolutely, unconditionally loving husband, and the miracle of healing. It was a miracle — a miracle in moving motion. It just took time, plenty of time, which I had an excess of then.

sixty-two steps

Another delicious experience occurred one day while in rehab, when the therapists challenged me by insisting I walk around the parallel bars while holding on to the orange vinyl table that stood elbow height. I played a game with myself: I'd hold on with my right hand, taking a few steps, then try to walk without holding on. Without realizing what I was doing, on this special day, I walked around the table without the use of my hand — taking 62 steps — all by myself! I became so excited, I phoned Norm on the way back to my room saying, "Guess what? I just took 62 steps — all by myself!" He cheered, and I could tell he was crying at the same time.

Another challenge I had was trying to use the pay phone and hospital bedside phone with my telephone credit card. I couldn't figure out how they worked. I felt foolish having to explain this to the operator, because I disliked having to admit my clumsiness and confusion. To this day, it's impossible to hold the phone in one hand and write a message. Norm finally installed a speakerphone at home to aid in this important function. He also placed a cushion onto the handset to rest on my shoulder. Any and all little technical aids like these make life easier and less frustrating.

the yellow-haired hallucination

During my excursions in the wheelchair when I was going to and from therapies, I had strange, almost hallucinatory experiences. I'd think I saw my former next-door neighbor, Mary S., who was a Registered Nurse and former hospital administrator. I thought she lived in Carmel, California. The last time I saw her she had been a brunette; now, in my stupor, she was a blond. Her image would appear to be sitting in various places throughout the hospital. One time she'd be sitting in one place; another time, she'd be in a different place (maybe a chair), in the corner of a hallway. As I'd wheel myself along the hallways, her image appeared like a ghost with yellow hair. I'd smile, and try to contact her; but there wouldn't be any response. I thought I was losing my mind, as well as my left side.

Fortunately, for my present-day sanity, I located evidence of this odd phenomenon in my research. "Reduplication delusions such as Capgras syndrome (the conviction that someone familiar has been replaced by an identical appearing impostor) has been observed following stroke and are more often associated with right than left hemisphere infarctions."[20]

---

[20] See Feinberg in the Bibliography for complete citation.

preparations for home

There would be various meetings throughout my hospital stay, called Case Conferences, with the hospital's primary team: physician, nurses, therapists, and family members. They structured themselves around my progress, which they evaluated during these meetings.[21] The time came after approximately two months of in-patient hospitalization to consider my return home.

> The average stay for in-patients eventually discharged home was nine to six weeks, while that for patients ultimately admitted to long stay accommodation was over 20 weeks. Some of the difference was due to the difficulty in arranging suitable long-stay care, some to the erroneous hope that prolonged intensive treatment in the Unit would eventually lead to a successful outcome.[22]

Eventually, the primary hospital doctor announced that, since I had declared my grief over not hearing the birds sing, my time to go home had come. I was walking by myself, with a cane, and felt more secure in this final challenge.

Preparations began: home visits by the proper therapists and social workers followed. They taught me how to close my eyes, eliminating one stimulus if I experienced too many stimuli, resulting in anxiety. This helped every time. It was like a mini-meditation. Dr. Sethi brought a lovely, large bouquet of flowers. I still see

---

[21] See Henley, et al. in the Bibliography.
[22] Journal of Neurology and Psychiatry, see Henly, et al. in the Bibliography for complete citation.

him standing at my door, holding the assorted arrangement, his turban as colorful as his fragrant farewell gift. It was a sensitive touch.

When it became necessary to determine who would be my home caregiver, I suggested using Mary S. — the "ghost" with yellow hair. It seemed like a natural idea. Norm placed a phone call to her and found she had recently moved her home from Carmel, California, to the Glendale area — close to our Studio City home. Was this another synchronicity? I asked myself if her appearance in the odd spots in the hospital could represent a figment of my imagination. Or could they create from actual planning? Or could they signify reality? Delusion? Fantasy? I don't recall the answer to that speculation.[23]

The reality of going home brought mixed feelings. For one, I couldn't wait, and confirmed this feeling by shouting "Hallelujah! Hooray! And howz about a right-handed high-five?" — all in one gulp. On the other hand, I would miss Susan, my faithful bedside room companion — as well as all the nurses and dedicated personnel.

the final farewell

I collected my mementos and memories, then sat in my wheelchair in the lighted hospital hallway, waiting for Norm and nurse Mary S. to tie up the loose ends. A favorite, wise, hospital staff nurse wished me well. She related a newspaper article she had recently read which told of a person who had a stroke and had gone back to school, receiving his doctorate. Inspiring, I thought. Inspiring . . .

---

[23] See Peroutka et al., Berthier, and Beckson in the Bibliography for complete citations.

wouldn't it be wonderful if I could achieve that! Yes, I pondered, looking down at Claw, wouldn't that be wonderful. The time had come for me to say good-bye to my hospital hassles, the first phase — and enter the reality of the real world. Enough about fantasy. Mary's car was waiting.

Chapter 9

HOME, MARY S. AND HER BEST GIFTS

my caregiver's teachings

MARY S. DROVE ME HOME; NORM RETURNED TO WORK. HE HAD A TV SHOW to tape that night. I rode in the passenger side of Mary's car feeling as though I had escaped from prison. We stopped for lunch in a sleazy, offbeat diner. It was the first time I ate non-hospital food. It tasted greasy. The daylight threatened my vision. It seemed brighter than usual; my eyes squinted from the glare.

After lunch, as we drove home, I noticed shadows playing gracefully on the surroundings. They looked symmetrical, artistic. It was as though I was seeing these familiar images for the first time. Springtime flirted with my emancipation. It was a paradox. I suddenly felt free, yet still harnessed in my new, unfamiliar confinement. I rolled down the window to hear my birds, to inhale the fresh air. The traffic frightened me. I noticed the Los Angeles smog, and began coughing to correct this impurity.

As my caregiver and as my attendant, Mary was indeed a gift. She showered me with daily baths and nourishing food, living in our home, teaching me how to dress, how to exist, and much more while Norm went to work. Her countenance possessed a spiritual quality with an aura and demeanor that taught me more about myself than I had ever learned previously. She was a protégée of the spiritual master, Brugh Joy, having attended most of his spiritual conferences. While she prepared meals, one among many of her gifts was sharing Brugh Joy's conference tapes on audio cassette. I listened with intrigue. Another transformational gift was reading his book (Joy's Way, 1979). These insights gently lifted me into a higher level of consciousness. One of his messages said: "There are no accidents." I knew this philosophy before, but for the first time I experientially felt these words and concept. Its meaning meant something. I was living this belief. Patricia Sun, a respected psychic healer, was also in Mary's circle of gurus. I listened to her healing sounds, meditating to her mystical melodies.

This phase was to be my awakening of the higher part of my unconscious, my soul; for Mary also taught me why my inner self called this stroke into my consciousness. That was a profound insight: a possibility that I actually called this stroke into my being. Therefore, I surmised, I had control over this bodily insult; albeit without my conscious knowing. I needed to ponder further for this understanding to manifest meaning.

Mary drove me to outpatient therapy at many different places: Glendale Adventist Hospital, Calabasas, back to Northridge Hospital for swimming therapy. I had acupuncture, range and motion therapy. We communicated in the car while she was driving; and while not driving. She taught me the Tao of Psychology,

Carl Jung, and every morning we used the Tarot cards introduced at my former graduate school as an access to one's unconscious. It was fascinating. I listened intently to her stories and inspiration and teachings. Norm began to think we were "weird."

Once, when Norm became irritated and intolerant from too much pressure, Mary summoned her innate wisdom: she and I fled in her car to her old, former home in Carmel, where we had a wild weekend holiday; a respite to clear the uneven air at home. When we returned, Norm seemed more relaxed, more tolerant, and much more able to cope with the severe loss that affected him as well. It was a brilliant strategy that Mary innocently planned, creating a much healthier atmosphere for all. I agreed heartily with the research I discovered that said, "the role of the counselor in the rehabilitation process is to help the stroke patient and his family learn to cope with the disability and to regain independence in their social-emotional functioning."

There was a natural ending to this phase. Mary had planned to attend another Brugh Joy conference in Hawaii, and had announced this plan earlier. I sensed the ending was coming, but felt sad to admit it was here. Mary was not only my caregiver, nurse, and attendant, but counselor, teacher, friend, and sister, sharing the same name as my real sister. When Mary left, my loss was deep, and I wept, sensing I was entering a new phase that beckoned. As a farewell gift, Mary gave me a crystal to hold in my right hand. It was a reminder of her energy, and mine, as well as my future — which was dawning.

Chapter 10

THE DARKNESS

isolation

MARY LEFT, AND I FELT LOST. I WAS ON MY OWN IN THIS STARK, DARK REALITY. Norm was working every day, including some weekends. All my friends worked. I had never been totally by myself, without a car or some means of transportation. We lived high in the Hollywood Hills, in a suburb called Studio City, nestled between Beverly Hills and the San Fernando Valley, located near Universal Studios. The compensation for this isolation was our Dona Teresa home. It was big and beautiful, with an oak-lined audio/video/editing booth Norm had designed on the fourth level. It looked out over the hills and the San Fernando Valley city lights. Our home served all the children when they lived with us. We had a view in three directions. It felt like being perched on top of a mountain summit, where hawks circle and glide, claiming their territory. Coyotes and other animals share this beauty with famous movie stars who live nearby. The roads are steep and narrow, with natural springs sometimes flooding the streets after a rainstorm. I decided I needed to make this my retreat, my island hideaway: a vacation, a refuge, until the next phase of this journey revealed itself.

synchronicities

It was like climbing from chaos to solitude — from hospital hassle to perfect paradise. I began to read many books of all kinds. Two experiences taught me synchronicity was in my realm. My plan was to read all my esteemed Uncle Rudolf Otto's books, which were on a spiritual plane. I had not managed to get through most of them before; they were highly esoteric and convoluted; the writing used in those days, I supposed. I knew he had coined the word numinous, which means finding the oneness with God in a spiritual sense. It is a mystical term Carl Jung used in his texts, giving credit to Otto.

I had put these books somewhere in our library bookshelf which was abundant with outstanding literature of all kinds. I could not find my uncle's books. I searched everywhere, for hours. This caused me great distress, for I felt that I had lost something very valuable again, which although unlike the "Ice" scissors, was certainly more useful and revered. I decided to forget the "compulsed" search, and began listening to John Bradshaw's audio tapes that a friend gave me.

When I had finished one side of tape #1, I said to myself, Wouldn't it be interesting if Bradshaw mentioned my uncle Rudolf. I turned the tape over, and the first thing Bradshaw said, on side #2, was to mention the valuable insights of Rudolf Otto. At that instant, I knew where his books were hiding, and marched directly to the cabinet, where I found them in back, on a bottom, dark shelf.

I pulled these dusty books from their mysterious hiding place and took them to my reading room. The first page that opened was a paragraph that mentioned exactly the same phenomenon that had just happened to me: finding something that you think you lost, and trusting the process that you will find it. It felt eerie, weird, strange, paranormal. It reminded me of the experience I had the night in the hospital, with stepson Shaun calling, as I explained earlier. Therefore, it was due to this heightened paranormal example that I knew I would find my lost self — if I relaxed and listened to my inner voice, trusting the process.

Everything from that point on flowed with my inner tuning.

I listened, put into practice many of Mary's teachings, and trusted my own lessons, for, as the quoted saying goes, "When the student is ready, the teacher appears." I was student, and teacher, to myself.

From that point, my daily focus included walking again in the hills, resuming my nature walks up and down the huge, steep hills, this time not bothered by my right eye going dark. However, in the morning my right hand was still sometimes numb. My inner teacher discovered the reason for that, which will reveal itself later. Suddenly, I remembered my father's two favorite coined sayings: #1, "Things will reveal themselves in time," and #2, "let nothing become commonplace." The first saying offers instant magic for the unfolding events that follow.

insights and lessons

Norm phoned me every day, just checking up to see how I was. I always sounded cheerful, occupying myself with my thoughts and own soap operas, stolen from my playful, and non-playful, prior phone friends. One was my aging mother who constantly complained about one thing or another. I listened. She had little tolerance for my condition, and didn't understand why this had happened to her daughter. This was a time, I later learned, for healing and achieving closure with her, for our years together never fully resulted in full acceptance of each other. We clashed painfully, each one stubborn and insensitive to the other's inner, innate energies. It was on her deathbed, literally, that I felt I had my final closure with her, when I activated peace with her demanding nature.

Another phone friend, Phyllis, who worked as a temporary worker, faithfully called me almost daily when she was not working. She'd share my grocery store salad that Norm had conscientiously made before he went to work; and when Phyllis would go on errands, often she invited me to go with her. This was a welcomed relief. We had the opportunity to share a friendship that I needed. I disclosed to her, one day while en route, that I felt envious of two-handed, working persons, for they had their independence — a condition I was trying to find. I am unaware if she understood my feelings.

The one daily pleasure that I looked forward to — which was about the only one other than my walks —was tuning in to Oprah Winfrey on TV at three o'clock. I planned all my phone calls, reading, and walks around this one activity. I dreamed of someday being on her show. The closest I got — so far — was seeing her in person at a taping at Universal Studios, where I sat on a hard, cold bench, surrounded by all the others in a multitude of faces. It was worth it. I saw in her brown eyes a sincerity that I admired as real. She was one of my inspirational, in-this-era, role models.

There was a day when I announced to Norm that I felt I just

couldn't function on my own anymore, and felt physically strange and drained inside. I didn't understand these feelings, and needed his help, again.

Chapter 11

DISCOVERING DEMONS, MEETING MONSTERS

THE DARKNESS OF THE DAWN STILL CONTINUED GETTING BLACKER AS THE HOURS passed. I was going to my outpatient physical therapies with my neighborhood barber, Mina, who lived across the canyon. I enjoyed her company, for she was kind and seemed eager to exchange dialogue as she drove. It was a new, growing friendship, fresh and fun, diverting me from my own self-absorption.

One of my therapists had had a stroke herself, and was improving rapidly. She said she couldn't wait to meet me, hearing how young I was. She had a great deal of strength in both her arms and hands so it was difficult accepting that she had such rapid recovery, or even had a stroke. Her story was an inspiration, and it felt comforting sharing this experience with someone like myself. We were birds of the same feather, like Siamese twins sharing the same soul.

At this particular rehab center I learned how to button my

shirts with easier control, given the helpful hint that by having someone sew elastic thread on the cuff buttons, I could get my hands into the sleeves much easier, because they stretched. It worked perfectly, and I use this device today.

Part of my research unearthed various strategies focusing on impairment training and task-specific training. These training approaches offer general and specific solutions to large and small problems. For example, it was suggested to keep rules simple because a patient's attention is often distractable and muddled in confusion, as was mentioned earlier.

a flashback

On Saturdays Norm dropped me off at my neighborhood manicurist, where I indulged in a manicure — a necessity, a simple pleasure. Keeping my fingernails shorter than I had in the past and avoiding bright polish was another loss I needed to resolve. One day when Norm dropped me off in the alley behind the salon, I watched as his car left slowly, headed in the direction of our home. As I watched his car disappear, suddenly I had a flashback that seemed to occur in breakneck, extraordinary speed. It went so fast I could not fathom the significance at the time it was happening. I put my right hand on the brass door knob of the salon, while simultaneously I saw myself as a very young child in my Alhambra bedroom, staring out of the window and watching my mother's green Chevrolet disappear down the street to nowhere.

She was driving it. I was alone, in my bedroom, getting ready for Janet's birthday party. Janet was my red-haired girlfriend who lived down the street, around the corner. I watched the clock carefully, knowing that when the "big hand reached the 12, the little hand on the two," I could leave, walking to her house. I felt sad because, before she left, my mother didn't tie my sash or give me a birthday present to take with me. I knew that presents were a requirement at someone's birthday party. What to do?

I decided, first of all, that it was impossible to tie my sash by myself so I let that go. As for a birthday present, I searched for my most favorite yarn doll and carefully moved a dining room chair in front of the hall cupboard. I climbed on top of the chair, standing on my tiptoes and reaching for a paper sack inside the cupboard. Having successfully found the smallest size, I wrapped my favorite yarn doll inside, making certain the paper sack rolled neatly without any wrinkles. I watched the clock, mindfully aware, until the proper time came; then I left on my walk to Janet's house. When I arrived at Janet's house, I stood on my tiptoes, again, ringing the doorbell. Mrs. Galbreath answered. I hurriedly explained my embarrassing plight, holding my carefully chosen paper sack in full view. She put her finger to her mouth, whispering, "Shhhh," spinning me around first, tying my sash, then taking my paper sack, and disappearing into her house, ushering me to find a place on the living room floor, where the other children were seated in a circle. When I saw the presents opening, I found Mrs. Galbreath had wrapped mine in paper, with pretty ribbon, and my sense of embarrassment faded.

As this flashback also faded, I found my hand back on the smooth brass doorknob at the salon, entering the building, confused, and feeling numb from this triggered memory. Norm returned to pick me up, and I told him this experience, which seemed unreal to both of us. I learned later, from remembering this experience, that when I'm feeling fearful I can recall the brass doorknob's smooth sensation and recollect this flashback, teaching myself: I can always take care of myself by figuring things out.

science-of-mind classes

During these days, my body was not feeling well. I had no energy when I awoke in the morning, finding it a chore to even climb out of bed; my menstrual periods were frequent, and heavy; also, my sleeping patterns simulated insomnia.

Yet somehow I managed to become inspired to attend Science-of-Mind classes at the Hollywood Church of Religious Science. These were weekly classes, preparing one to become a Science-of-Mind practitioner and healer. The minister/teacher of these classes, Domenic Polifrone, was a motivating speaker, and he filled me with determination and euphoria. I seemed to inhale all of his inspiration and theory. His presence was charismatic. I found myself enchanted by the philosophy that people could influence their lives by what they thought. In other words, people can sculpt their thinking by attitude and action, by employing affirmations. It was like my visualizing Homecoming Queen years earlier. I became a true believer and active participant. Norm drove me to the classes; someone in the group drove me home. "Where there's a will; there's a way" — right in keeping with Science-of-Mind thinking.

I affirmed for my energy to improve and to feel better physically. This desire became so intense, I made an appointment with our neighborhood physician to give me every test available, from Auto Immune Deficiency Syndrome, to whatever. I was determined to feel well.

Dr. Freeman's results were revealing. The blood tests indicated

I had Epstein-Barr, candida, and arsenic poisoning! I couldn't believe it: but, it was true.

All these strange conditions happened at the same time. No wonder I could barely get out of bed. From the blood tests Dr. Freeman speculated that the high level of arsenic came from eating too much unwashed spinach — along with pesticides — in the vegetable salads from our local market. Norm made new fresh salads every day for my lunch before he went to work.

a cleansing

This was another low time for me, as the cure from all these meant I needed medical treatment in Dr. Freeman's office with daily Vitamin C intravenous solutions, multivitamin therapy, as well as well as colonics. This treatment plan was used to cleanse my intestines — as if I hadn't had enough from my previous hospital stay! This therapy did work, for eventually I recovered with more energy.

It was somewhere around this time in my healing process that Norm and I took a one-week respite in Hawaii to cleanse our souls from this past nightmare. I recall we traveled with an extra suitcase — primarily loaded with various bottles of vitamins, herbs and amino acids. When I put all of the bottles out on the hotel dresser, they completely covered the entire surface. I saw the confused look on the house cleaner's face when she saw this assortment of bottles. She probably thought we were drug abusers!

This was a strange vacation. I recall my body was razor thin — not something that I minded — mirroring the unhealthy state I was in. We spent most of our days inside the hotel room reading. We were quiet, rarely talking, which was unusual for "our dance."

Something under the surface was brewing, but I couldn't put my finger on it. We had been to Hawaii many times, together and separately.

It triggered a memory I experienced a month after I returned home from Northridge Hospital. I traveled with Judy. We went to spend a week with Diane on Kauai. I recall how nervously anxious I was. In the airport, many stimuli surrounded me: colors, sights, sounds — stimuli buzzing. I was not accustomed to them, at that raw time, which confused and bothered me. That's when I put into practice closing my eyes, blocking out one too many stimuli, acting like a mini-meditation. Judy was a magnificent friend, helping me at every corner: unpacking my suitcase, cutting my meat, buttering my bread, helping me to dress and undress, comforting my fears, talking to me, not making me feel ashamed for my feelings. Also, she even attached onto my back, the TENS (a pain-relieving) machine. It was the last time I needed the help of that marvelous pain-control machine as the pain vanished in my back and shoulder area forever.

Nevertheless, when I was with Norm on our vacation this Kauai reverie simulated feelings I had with my girlfriends — my graduate school colleagues. Perhaps it was from inhaling the fragrant plumeria which revived the memories with them, when Norm and I were in our quiet moods.

Nothing appeared faulty on the surface, and as time smoothed out this adventure, it proved to be merely a quiet, reflective, pensive time for both. I surmised that we each needed to be in our separate caves. Soon we fell back on track, ready for the next challenge, which greeted us shortly after returning home.

Chapter 12

A Crack of Light Appears

UCLA and NPI

MY PHYSICAL BODY HAD IMPROVED FROM THE EARLIER LOSS OF ENERGY, BUT THERE would be moments when my body still felt as though it couldn't function. The "little engine that could," couldn't. I announced that feeling to Norm, and he said, "We've tried everything. The last resort is UCLA." I thought this was an excellent idea — UCLA being so close to our home — and a teaching university as well.

We made an appointment for an evaluation, being admitted immediately to their NPI (Neuropsychiatric Institute). This was to be the second most enlightening phase in my healing — the first was Northridge Hospital.

Following admittance, I existed behind locked doors, where searching and frisking are mandatory. It was like being in a movie where they search for concealed weapons on the person. I felt insulted by this; however, I understood the reason after a strange person came into the shower room and rummaged through my cosmetic bags. Finally, they put me into my own small bedroom, directly across from the woman's bathroom. My bedroom was as big as my walk-in closet at home, with the closet being half the size of a coffin.

I had numerous roommates. The first one was manic, who would suddenly terrorize me by running up and down the outside hallway in the middle of the night. The nightly custom was to stuff a washcloth in between the door and the door frame, in order to keep the door slightly ajar. The theory for this was to keep the door from banging when the night nurse opened it to observe our sleeping patterns.

This technique was disturbing. After quietly opening the door, the night nurse would shine a flashlight onto my face to see whether or not I was asleep. This monitoring usually disturbed me, whether I was sleeping or awake. My sleeping patterns were becoming disturbed more frequently.

I was aware of them using direct observation on me, during the day and during the nighttime, by the nurses and the physicians. My primary doctor was a female by the name of Pamela Summit.

When she interviewed me I commented on her name by saying she had obviously reached the summit. There was an absence of laughter, absence of a smile; not even a small tittering or twinkles in her eyes. Although I created this corny comment for connection, I had the feeling she was serious, dedicated, and businesslike. I didn't expect her to be "Ms. Santa Claus," but I could have used some humor. Nevertheless, I restrained this need until Norm could find me again, after his work. He always provoked laughter with his natural humor.

When I stated my physical problems to Dr. Summit, I had previously planned for this assessment by taking a yellow legal pad and listing one by one the journey of my illness and complaints. I wanted to be accurate, concise, determined to regain my normal state of health. I felt embarrassed when I read this list, for it covered a page and a half. I thought for certain she would diagnose me as a hypochondriac.[24] All she needed to do, however, was verify my list by my other former physicians, which eventually she did.

This entire UCLA process was an experience I would never trade. I felt as though it was a living, experiential adventure in the midst of the medical/mental health field. How many of my future colleagues would experience living as a patient in a psychiatric care facility? During my current research I sought evidence that this type of training, — being a psychotherapist and a patient in an inpatient psychiatric setting — offered value, and an edge to the psychotherapist's training. However, I was unable to document this data, even though I have heard about the significance of this experience. Consequently, this inability to locate and document this information caused me great distress, as I know the experiential value to be worth more than any university/textbook training.

bizarre behavior

I observed the various people who shared this theater with me: from homeless, delusional types to those who appeared catatonic, schizophrenic, manic, bipolar, with depression symptoms; to obsessive-compulsive disorders, exhibiting red hands, raw from washing.

[24] See Newman in the Bibliography.

I fit in there, too, with my burgeoning compulsiveness, beginning to exhibit bizarre behavior by my hoarding strange things like tampons, in case I had a "gusher" unexpectedly (which happened many times, leaving me incapacitated and embarrassed, with the use of only one hand to handle the emergency). I didn't like seeing the red spot on my jeans, which usually shrunk when they were washed, making them impractical and impossible to try to fit into again and fasten with one hand.

I felt also bothered by my sudden impulse to shoplift silly, unimportant things like earrings, which I could well afford to pay for. It is an embarrassing behavior pattern to admit, for that was most unusual compared to my past behavior pattern. From my schooling, I learned it is not unusual for a right hemisphere, brain-impaired person to manifest this uncontrolled, spontaneous, impulsive behavior marked by changed, radical deviations from previous past behavior. I am thankful for my education! I wondered why the hospital personnel had failed to apprise me of this shameful, horrifying characteristic. That was one of the major reasons for admitting myself to this institution.

There were all the textbook categories of mental illness: serious, hard-core mental illnesses that were interesting to study, from my curious, nonprofessional standpoint.

drugged and dazed

It appeared that almost all the inmates in this unit were on drugs. They would walk around in a glazed, stupor state. After my own personal, direct observations were finished, as well as the medical team's observance of my reactions, I fell into the drugged group as well.

When Dr. Summit learned I had Takayasus Disease, she summoned the entire medical force at UCLA to observe me. At one point, the doctors assembled in the auditorium, with me on center stage, each one examining me with stethoscopes tethered to their necks; each one poking, prodding, prying into, onto my chest and limbs. At one point I counted 32 faces; 32 white jackets; 32 stethoscopes, and over 100 questions. I could have written a song, entitled, "32 Doctors, 100 Questions!" And, there were comments such as: "You're so young to have this rare disease;" "I think you must be in remission."

I didn't like that word: remission. I told these doctors that my right hand was still numb in the morning; yet their tests and examinations found nothing — nothing! They didn't bother sleuthing it out, like a detective looking for clues.

After the medical team concluded direct observations they prescribed Trazodone[25] (Deseryl), the sedative antidepressant, that produced a frightening effect. Not only did it cause extreme incontinence, which meant I didn't make it to the toilet in time (experiencing a wet bottom); but also, while eating, without warning, my head would slump and fall on the table in the dining room, hitting it with a thud. "You'll get used to the dosage," the authorities said. I don't think I ever did, and was consumed by fear: fear that I would fall in my unbalanced stupor. I needed to be careful as my left leg was highly unsteady. I needed all the help I could get.

a true test

The authorities also gave me another battery of tests, similar to

---

[25] See Reding, et al. in the Bibliography.

those given at Northridge Hospital, except this time it included the Minnesota Multiphasic Personality Inventory. Curious, I was never apprised of the results. The day we were to begin, I began bleeding profusely and had to terminate the test; for it was a messy, embarrassing situation. The examiner understood, and we resumed later.

Another infamous day included my old graduate school friend Diane, and my other old Whittier College roommate, Frida. They came to visit me. It was a happy surprise. They brought with them the most outstanding, enormous, colorful bouquet of flowers I had ever seen, equipped with a marbleized vase as well. It took four hands to hold it. I took one look at their piece of artwork, and realized immediately the love involved. They told the story of hand-picking these flowers, traipsing in bare feet in a meadow with sprinklers on, collecting the multicolored variety themselves. It was a comical, cute story that brought tears to my eyes, for I could visualize their drama, viewing the love in their eyes; their hearts, their pride evident, expressed colorfully, artistically, honestly. When I brought the heavy bouquet to my bedroom, the staff made me get rid of it. I wilted. I felt crushed. Their rule was: no one can have a container of glass or breakable substance. It's too easy for someone to break the vase in order to slash their wrists.

I felt as though I was in prison again. I was ready to slash my wrists — or someone's — after they forced me to destroy the bouquet. My heart broke, and I was ready to show that I could indeed have a tantrum in public. Refraining was a true test of patience.

In occupational therapy, I tried to get control of myself by relaxing. The therapists insisted I work on some kind of project. It was one of their rules. I decided to make a wooden board, with two nails inserted in the center, to use as a one-handed cutting board. This required me to sandpaper the board with an electric sander, using my right hand. After working on this for a substantial period of time, I managed not only to injure my right arm from so much sanding, resulting in a cramping, but this also affected my back, which ached for days, requiring Norm to bring my cane so I could reinstate the use of it. I hobbled like an old person. This board remains on top of my refrigerator today, as a helpful idea when needed, albeit a painful reminder that I must take care of Claw's friend.

scenes from a film

One of the outdoor activities was marching with a group of inmates onto the streets of Westwood with Nurse Armstrong in the lead. We'd pass students coming and going to their classes, until ending up on the athletic field, where I'd walk as fast as I could feeling like a hamster in a treadmill: round and round I'd go. I told Nurse "Strongarm," as I'd call her, that I felt like one of the gang in the movie, "One Flew Over the Cuckoo's Nest." She noted it in my chart. I just wasn't certain who played the role of Jack Nicholson, or Nurse Ratchet.

When I was back in my closetlike room overlooking the city of Westwood, I'd feel sad, remembering when I had exhibited my artwork in The Westwood Art and Craft Show and did so well. I could almost see the spot where my stand was, and where my friends would come, supporting my wares and whims. Nurse Strongarm thought I felt depressed; I may have been, as a post-bereavement reaction. I cried frequently. Moreover, it felt like a grief reaction to me — a premenstrual sensation, similar to Premenstrual Syndrome.

One night I awoke in a pool of blood. Alarmed, I walked bare-footed to the nurse's station to tell the night nurse. She told me to wait until morning when the doctor would be available. Therefore, I hid in the woman's bathroom trying to take care of myself — with one hand. The ugly truth was, when I left, the stall appeared to look like a brutal bloody murder had occurred.

Early in the morning, I was in a chair by the nurses' station, waiting. I looked up and saw Dr. Summit enter the double doors. She bent down to tell me she needed to rearrange our afternoon appointment. I quickly interrupted her, saying I was hemorrhaging, severely. She said, "Oh, my God," and immediately called for a wheelchair and attendant who, before I could say my name, rushed me down to the OB-GYN clinic. In my mind there is a grisly, graphic picture of what really happened. I hesitate painting this appalling portrait; however, its importance ties in with my later discovery, and recovery. It is like a scene from an inhuman horror film, but worse.

I waited again, what seemed like an eternity, spilling blood along the floor, leaving a trail, even with thick sweatpants on. This description seems ugly to write, although its depiction documents in a literal fashion, without deletion, the torture I endured, however ugly, gory, and graphic. The drama was chilling to me, wanting to be modest at all times in my demeanor. Perhaps that explains my original compulsion: hoarding tampons, not wanting to be caught in this embarrassing predicament.

They gave me a biopsy. Later, the Chief of the Gynecology Department told me that I was "in the middle of menopause" but, because I had periods, the menopause was "incomplete." He prescribed estrogen. The other doctors who conferred disagreed, saying that because I'd had a stroke, it was dangerous to give me estrogen. They prescribed progesterone instead.

my mission

I went back to my bedroom and resumed the activities that occupied my days. One of the most satisfying experiences was talking to the inmates there. We seemed to have a jolly time, forming our own spontaneous clique, despite the incarceration. One of the people was the grandson of the museum billionaire, Norton Simon. He was elf-like: funny, entertaining, and clever, but bipolar. I also became friendly with a depressed person, Inez, initially a bland, petite person, who was originally from Ecuador, South America. We communicated for hours. During this exchange, I gave her information on the principles of Science-of-Mind. When she heard this, as well as observing my claw condition, it created a major change in her life. She accepted this philosophy and, within a short amount of time, blossomed. She began applying make-up, and after her release called to tell me she bought a red dress! She also planned her time around her Science-of-Mind studies. When they released me, we continued to communicate. She wrote lovely, expressive letters, penmanship perfect, thanking me for being her channel. I believe if I had not entered this institution, Inez would have remained a lost soul, never having been saved. Although narcissistic in relating this, I have kept her letters as evidence that a seed had been planted in fertile soil — or hungry soul — which helped heal another valuable human being. That was only one of the many healing experiences with which I felt connected.

I went to group therapy with others who were greedy for answers. I spoke to an obsessive-compulsive person — whose hands were red and raw from washing so frequently — just before he went home. After listening to him and relating to his story, I received his blessing. He said no one had helped him "see the light" as I had done. Claw gave him hope. The counselors told me that my calling was in helping others; my spirit seemed to radiate healing. However, a certain nurse instructed me to "cool it" for I was not a "professional." Miraculously, I realized my mission in life, and thanked Claw. Helping others is indeed my calling. A crack of light became visibly apparent, at last!

Chapter 13

THE SEARCHLIGHT

medication monitoring

WHEN I LEFT UCLA TO RETURN TO MY HOME, THE QUIET SANCTUARY, I FELT lonely for the members of the clique that had formed such a strong support feeling, while under the care of the numerous doctors and nursing staff. The inmates may have been ill, but I felt a powerful connection with everyone. This had been a deep bond.

Following my hospital treatment, I was instructed by the UCLA doctors to seek the care of a county psychiatrist to monitor my medication, Deseryl. I also disliked being on medication, and vowed to get off, with the proper physician.

I had a horribly frightening experience getting off amitriptyline, prescribed in Northridge Hospital, mentioned earlier. To reiterate: when I felt I was ready to quit amitriptyline, I told Dr. King. He said, "Okay, just cut the pills in half." I did that, and when the dosage became reduced, I felt as though I was going insane and wanted to bang my head against a wall.[26]

I discovered later in my Psychopharmacology class at school that this type of harmful, inaccurate reduction can create high anxiety. Not understanding the term anxiety at that time, I must have experienced it unknowingly, inappropriately labeling the feeling insanity for anxiety. At odd moments, I would approach Norm, asking him to "please, just hold me." I needed him to hold me, I'd emphasize. He'd hold me, but I still felt strange in my head. Thus, I sought a private psychiatrist, Dr. Zackler, who said it was dangerous to "cut the pills in half." One never could get the exact equal dosage. Therefore, he reduced my dosage, gradually, slowly, which resulted in no more of the acute anxiety or symptomatic feelings that left me feeling as though I were going insane. Also, he put me with one of his interns for brief therapy. I must have been in denial; for after several sessions, I felt bored, choosing to discuss the latest, current books with her instead of my symptoms.

However, the reduction of the medication, gradually, was a hard lesson I needed to learn. Recently, I found audiotapes of these sessions, evidence proving how really depressed I seemed. Insight from my recent education at school indicates I must have suffered a slight memory loss problem as well — not recalling this sadness or depression. It was interesting to note that "memory is rarely assessed in studies of stroke patients."[27]

Still, the county psychiatrist, Dr. Gurman, had my medical history and reduced my Deseryl dosage, gradually, with no after effects. It was an easy transition, and after completely going off Deseryl, I didn't feel depressed. I felt as I did before — almost normal. The pieces in the puzzle were coming together.

---

26 See Messner and Messner in the Bibliography for a complete citation.
27 See Lincoln, et al. in the Bibliography for complete citation.

the mystery is solved

Another post-UCLA instruction was to seek an outside OB-GYN doctor in my area. My former GYN specialist had retired, so I took the recommendation from the Chief of Gynecology at UCLA, a Dr. Pearson.

After hearing my extensive medical history, Dr. Pearson, in his thick English accent, told me was going to take a risk. Despite the hesitations from the UCLA gynecology specialists, he put me on estrogen patches, which were "milder than the pill form," he added.

The minute I began this replacement therapy, I felt like a different person. Overnight my mood and physical body felt totally different: I felt alert, active, clear-headed, less irritable, less anxious, and I slept at night. No more insomnia. No more embarrassing bloodied beds. I was a different person. It was as though someone had raised a curtain — the veil lifted. A new person was born.

I saw things differently. I heard things differently. I felt things differently. It was another wonderful hallelujah, hooray, and amen! I was ready for action, ready for stimulation. I wondered why all the 32 doctors, plus, who were absent at the auditorium's examination, didn't put two and two together, diagnosing me as a typical menopausal person. A determined detective would have succeeded with more accurate results. My age was right; my symptoms in perfect conformity to the textbook theories.[28] It made me question the integrity and abstract thinking of the medical profession. My trust in this large teaching university faded, but not my memories. They were vivid.

---

28 Refer to Gail Sheehy's The Silent Passage: Menopause for a more complete description.

I was ready to search out new stimulation, ready to learn more from life. Someone switched on my searchlight, and I scouted the territory, like an archeologist, unearthing a dig for a significant find. The menu was vast, the choices varied.

the stroke support group

Unable to drive, I had Norm take me to a stroke support group held at the Presbyterian Hospital in Van Nuys.

I was comfortable with my fellow sufferers, who shared more than handicap placards. On my first visit, I met Jim, who had been unable to talk for eight years. What a nightmare, I thought. Eight years! His spouse sat beside him, talking for him. Another young person, Marty — same name as mine — had suffered several strokes from a faulty heart valve. She was a single person with much courage and spirit. Another person, Dick, had a stroke, which authorities assumed because he was obese. His spouse Judith was his faithful, constant companion, always close at hand. Another person, Marvin, also couldn't talk. His spouse Cookie, constantly looking as colorful as my computer's screen saver and as stylish as a model, was peppy and helpful. She also stayed beside her spouse, but encouraged him to talk for himself.

Others were sitting around the circle, some in wheelchairs, some in the metal chairs next to the brown tables. Some had white hair, some black, some blond, some balding. A few, with right-hemisphere injuries like myself, cried, unable to quiet themselves. Usually there would be some event that we shared, like a movie, or listening to an informative speaker; refreshments followed. It became a social affair to which I looked forward. Yet, I didn't want to be identified with this group. I felt like a snob at times, feeling I was different; however, knowing inside I wasn't different, because Claw was there to remind me. Although not always humble, I learned humility.

Once there was a speaker at the meeting — a Doctor of Psychology, Dr. Backarack — who spoke about the realities of having had a stroke, although he had not had one. He encouraged us to have pet names for our paralyzed limbs. I had already named my hand Claw, so I called my leg Stump, for that's what it felt like. Now Claw had a buddy with which to relate.

Dr. Backarack also conducted hypnosis, which intrigued me. Maybe, I thought, I could overcome my handicap by hypnosis. I put this under consideration for later.

At another Stroke Club meeting, there was a new member, a former attorney named Ted. He was a bright, handsome young person, the father of small children. He came with his petite spouse, and they sat quietly, apart from others I presumed, because he could not talk. I watched him maneuver himself awkwardly in his wheelchair, cautiously. After listening to the others share, he began to try to speak, painfully aware of his hollow, grunting sounds that sputtered and stammered slowly. We all were respectfully quiet when he began speaking. He said he could not work anymore as an attorney; therefore, he retired and took up novel writing on his computer. He had cranked out several books, which he had published, and was working on another. He said, "The stroke was the best thing that ever happened to me."

I sat stunned hearing this. How, I thought, could the stroke be the best thing that ever happened to anyone? It mystified me, but in his testimonial, I saw an inner peace reflecting behind his eyes that told me he was finally a happy person, who originally disliked law practice, and used this crisis to turn his life around. He changed in one instant. I became inspired by his story, leaving that meeting with a different attitude.[29]

Another club meeting found everyone sharing, as usual, along with a new member who told his story. At the end, he disclosed he could not hold his grandchild, which he never considered would ever happen. When I heard that, I broke down in deep sobs, for it was something that I never considered either. When it became my turn to hold my first grandchild last year, this man's story recalled my grief then, and I cried again, while holding my first grandbaby, Jessica, for the first time — with a pillow supporting my right arm. While rocking her in the hospital room's rocking chair, I whispered my feelings to her, hoping she would be patient with me, and love me for who I was inside, not what physically manifested. I will learn the results of this whispered request in time.

Norm shared with me his amazement while watching me still sleeping in the morning after he awoke. He sometimes would see Claw opening; slowly stretching, uncurling its spasticity, becoming pliable, almost normal, compared to its fetal, tightly clenched fist. I was not privy to this remarkable event, and also marveled at the possibility that normalcy was returning. Perhaps Norm's continual nightly efforts at giving me my range and motion physical therapy was making the neurons click into orbit, or function, again. It was hope, and we both remembered Dr. Backarack's tempting invitation of hypnosis.

hypnosis

We decided to try hypnosis. We had nothing to lose, except

---

[29] See Thompson, et al. in the Bibliography.

$80 a session. Dr. Backarack's office was in Beverly Hills. Norm would leave work early and take me on this special trip, over the hill from our home.

I relaxed into Dr. Backarack's chair, accepting his suggestions for four sessions. There was no improvement. I felt disappointed, but learned from my Physiology class in school that, once injured, the neurons in the brain are dead and will not rejuvenate, merely forming new pathways to compensate. I found a case study,[30] along with education that visualization, guided imagery exercises help the stroke patient relax, thus improving their condition and lessening pain; but because of the rationale that the immutable effects of brain damage cannot be disputed, or denied — even though new neural associations form until death, and compensatory development functions — sadly and unfortunately, hypnosis does not aid in this neurological miracle of restoration. (It is also interesting to note that Holroyd's credentials indicate she is associated with the Neuropsychiatric Institute of California at Los Angeles — NPI!)

further healers

This did not stop our efforts towards a physical miracle. Norm had learned at work through an office employee, Barbara, that there was a healer in the Hollywood neighborhood who had helped her with an illness. It was worth another try.

We went to this person, who made no claims at healing, for he was as mystified as everyone else who received benefit. He would place his hands over my body, while I rested on a hard, narrow

---

[30] See Holroyd in the Bibliography.

table. I could actually feel warmth radiating from his hands, as they hovered above me. On one occasion, suddenly, I manifested a lump, the size of a golf ball, which appeared on my left upper arm. Associated with this lump was a sharp pain. This was highly unusual. My entire left side from head to toe was without feeling. I cried out in agony. The pain was like a charley horse in the arm. It took several days for the lump to disappear, as well as the pain, but there was no direct improvement to Claw. We terminated these sessions after I showed no progress.

However, we remain forever open to every avenue, every hope, every variety of healing, including prayer, for we want Claw and Stump to restore their original form.

sharing sorrow and stages of spouses

On one particular Sunday, Norm and I decided to attend the activity expo for physically challenged people at the LA Convention Center. It had a crowded array of booths and exhibits demonstrating the newest and latest items in the handicapped world — from creative clothes to newfangled wheelchairs, to art work by an artist who painted with his toes. As we were combing the aisles, we spotted the stroke support group people, in a cluster, examining a booth. I had not seen them for a short period of time; therefore, it was a hometown, small world, friendly feeling to find them. I saw everyone in our circle, except Dick. I asked his spouse, Judith, where he was. "He died," she announced abruptly, bursting into tears. Stunned, I broke into wailing sobs of sympathy, sharing her pain. It was another sad moment that required healing. It put a damper in the group's expo-exploration, and we sensed it was time to leave.

I drove home with Norm in pensive contemplation, reaching over the car's console, needing his comfort, his consolation. I felt he did likewise. We touched hands in silence. I thought, perhaps Dick was better off, and Judith was too. I couldn't adjust to this thought as I studied Norm's profile while he drove. A strokee's mate is as important to her as her own breathing.

In all of my research the repetitive mention of importance of spouse is cited. Although some studies indicate that single patients may survive better than married patients do, generally it can be stated "having a spouse is a very important determinant."[31] Moreover, findings expound on the reduction in social contact with patients and spouses, as well as lessening of leisure activities. I found a characterization of the stages[32] that the spouses of stroke patients may proceed through, which includes the period of hospitalization:

Stages

Stage 1 Crisis and shock: this occurs when the patient is taken to hospital.

Stage 2 Hope and anxiety: the patient shows some signs of recovery and although the family is anxious that death may occur, they do have some hope of a recovery.

Stage 3 Relief and concern switch: it is now clear that the patient will not succumb and attention is directed towards the treatment and recovery.

[31] See Lincoln in the Bibliography.
[32] See Newman in the Bibliography.

Stage 4 Increased expectations: the family's expectations of a full recovery are increased as the recovery continues.

Stage 5 Homecoming: all attention is directed towards this event, seen by the family as another milestone on the path to full recovery.

Stage 6 Maintenance of expectations: as the patient continues to improve expectations of a full recovery are maintained.

Stage 7 Doubts and concerns: the patient's rate of progress declines and the family becomes concerned as to whether the anticipated full recovery will occur.

Stage 8 Realization: the family now realizes that little improvement will occur and that they now have to cope with the patient in the present state.

Elizabeth Kubler-Ross refers to five stages of growth during terminal illness: "following Health (Stability) is when the terminal illness is diagnosed (which creates a significant charge). Stage I: Denial (Shock); this generates loneliness, internal conflict, guilt, meaninglessness, resulting in Stage II: Anger (Emotion); which leads to Stage III: Bargaining (gradual realization of the real consequences); Stage IV: Preparatory (Depression), then followed by Movement toward self-awareness and contact with others. Finally, this points to Stage V: Acceptance (increased self-reliance)."

self magazine and synchronicity

Another stage, or phase, was silently budding. One afternoon, while in the privacy of my downstairs bathroom, I picked up a current *Self* magazine and thumbed through unread articles. There was one that leaped out at me immediately. Its title was, "The Changing American Family." I thought, I know all about this from my graduate studies, and did not need to read it.

Yet, this instant popping out of the page reminded me of something — almost like a flashback or déjà vu. It reminded me of a time when my friend Frida and I attended a lecture, in an Altadena library, on some subject that interested us. While I felt mesmerized by the speaker's talk, my Uncle Rudolf Otto's image came to me, again. I asked Frida to accompany me to the restroom so I could recover from this unusual specter. On our way, we rounded a corner in the library's lined row of books, stumbling on a book in the aisle that had fallen from a shelf. Frida picked it up. It was *Mysticism East and West* by Rudolf Otto! Frida and I looked at each other in disbelief, for she was aware of the stature of my uncle's reputation. She did not know my concurrent thought until I told her, however. We both felt chills from the experience.

Consequently, this flashback centered me quickly, and as that thought planted itself in my mind, my inner voice spoke in heady words, commanding me to read that Self magazine article. I read the article. It spoke about some details that I already knew from graduate studies about the family realm; but it went deeper, with empathic stories describing various places where people were helping people: retirement areas — in particular, Leisure World in Laguna Hills, California, that specialized in caregiving service for the elderly and the handicapped. It told of having a transportation system, plus over 200 clubs and organizations in every type and kind of activity. My eyes grew wide with wonderment and enthusiasm. It sounded like a place where I would like to live: paradise! Being a native Californian, I had always wanted to live in the Newport Beach/Laguna area, because of its perfect climate.

I eagerly confronted Norm about my discovery, becoming like a child, more excited the more I spoke about it. He said, "Sounds interesting. Call for information and literature." Usually I left things like that up to him, but this time I took him up on the offer, phoning immediately. Within a week, we received a packet of inviting information. We made arrangements to take their grand tour.

We both fell in love with Leisure World instantly. I couldn't wait to put our home up for sale. The problem was that Norm was still working, and we needed the money to survive. Our hospital bills were enormous. I had trouble tethering my emotions; my enthusiasm was obvious. I wanted this move to happen, yesterday! I felt ready to engage in the real world again.

a stern reaction and rejection

Often we took my mother out to dinner. In her aging process she was becoming more resentful, cranky, and complaining, especially about Doc — the grumpy pharmacist. She was living her life in uneasy despair, realizing she had made a terrible mistake in marrying him, as he embarrassed her in every situation: from cruise ship dinners to San Marino social events. Each had paid a price for their unfortunate marriage. One evening, following our out-to-dinner treats, I couldn't resist sharing my Leisure World discovery with her. I blurted out the fabulous feelings I had, and all the glory associated with this community — being perfect for Norm and me in my present reality. Her first comment, after hearing our future plans was "Why do you want to do a stupid thing like that?"

I became quiet, excusing myself, distancing myself again from this abuse. I went to the bathroom, feeling the inner sadness creep up, choking my ability to talk back. "Don't you dare talk back, Martha Jane, or you'll get your mouth washed out with soap." These were the words I had heard from her since I could first remember, maybe when two years old. I had the cleanest mouth in the neighborhood. Thinking back, I always felt anger and sadness, from cruel comments such as this, even at an early age.

Writing this stimulates the memory of an incident which occurred in our laundry room, on the back porch, arguing about something. I was about 13 years old at the time. She yelled at me, "I'm going to tell the man you marry what a horrible person you are!" With this, I shut my mouth, again, secretly knowing there was a good person inside waiting to express herself to someone who would listen. It was obvious, I couldn't talk back; therefore, we never could communicate because I was unable to talk back; she was unable to listen.

There were comments or affronts such as these as recently fresh as two weeks prior to this visit: "Why can't my daughter do the laundry?" She said this, after Norm had announced we needed to leave her home earlier than expected one evening, because he was in the middle of doing our laundry. Fortunately Norm had a way with her mean-spirited nature, and simply smiled his beautiful smile, saying, "But, Hazel, I prefer to do it myself." She could say or do nothing but nod.

When I returned from the bathroom after her put-down on my stupidity for wanting to move to Leisure World, I rested my case. In my quietness, she tried to resume her battle by saying, "You don't love me. You never did." I kept silent, as I'd been instructed to do at two years old. I'd let her have her way, one more time, knowing how I felt inside. I would have liked to have said, "Yes, you're right, I never did love you; you wouldn't let me." But there was no point. It didn't matter. It was too late.

mother's death

Mother died at age 88, shortly after this last attempt to control me. As she lay on her deathbed I managed to listen to her life's recriminations. I blew her a kiss, as I left her bedside for the last time, telling her that I loved her and would see her in another life. But I know in my heart, in the next life, I will be master of myself — or maybe be my own mother, as well. I certainly was my own mother in this life.

An interesting footnote in this sad, bittersweet story should be told. My parents had a gentle caregiver living in their San Gabriel house, named Claire. She related to me that prior to Hazel's death, an aging neighbor came to their front door, inquiring how Doc and Hazel were. Claire and this elderly gentleman remarked how mentally sharp Doc still was at 96 years old. The neighbor's comment was, "Yes he is, and the only sharp thing about Hazel is her tongue." After hearing this, I congratulated myself for enduring her abuse. I wasn't the only person who felt this way about her mean spirit. His comment was like a final verification that I wasn't wrong — after all those years.

We cleaned out their house, following Doc's demise at 98. It was a painful parting in some respects; in other ways, it was a true cleansing for me, a final freeing. Our family helped dispose of much of the lifelong clutter, giving it to less fortunate people who needed it. I salvaged a few nostalgic mementos for the descendants. Friends of ours, Barbi and Jack Crosby — Jack being the nephew of Bing Crosby — became involved in the sorting of the stuff. They have a small business that buys and sells garage sale items. They were instrumental in deciding which were valuable, and which were worthless.

valuable insights

I found myself at home experiencing strange reactions following mother's death. As an example, once, when I dropped something accidentally, I heard a voice inside say, "What did you do that stupid thing for, you clumsy kid?" Then, I'd say, "It's okay. You didn't mean to do it." Then, I'd take my right arm and hug myself. It was a self-comforting, reparenting feeling that felt naturally healing.

Even today, if Norm becomes impatient with me, or gives the slightest indication of displeasure, speaking harshly, or is critical, I snap right back into that past mind frame of mother's scoldings. It goes deep within.

While we were in San Francisco on holiday at Christmastime a few years ago, we were in an exclusive department store with Norm's brother, Tony. They were going to go to another department in the store, so Norm told me to sit down in a chair in the shoe section, where I could wait for them. As they left Norm said, "I'll be back," and, as a whispered aside, added, "if you're lucky." When I heard him say this, even though intellectually I knew it was intended to be a dumb joke, I burst into tears, which streamed down my face. I felt silly sitting in a shoe department sobbing, but the impact of this feeling of abandonment was a deep hurt, which later I translated from my little girl feeling abandoned at a small age: to mother driving away in the green Chevrolet, to Daddy leaving me — forever — at eight years old, which was also a factor. Mother's obvious lifelong abandonment through noncommunication was a reason as well. This abandonment issue is being resolved now, partially due to Norm's realization and patience. Now he says, "I'm going to my cave - but, I'll be back." This was a helpful hint learned from John Gray's book: *Men are from Mars, Women are from Venus* — a useful guide for my plight.[33]

Following mother's death, my inheritance enabled us to put our huge house up for sale, with the intention of moving to Leisure World in Laguna Hills. Norm was without work, as it was becoming apparent after a long, extensive work search that the more mature workers (referred to in the television industry as "gray-heads") were being phased out, discriminated against. There was much controversy on the subject, seen in the news, written in newspapers and in magazine reviews. After his successful career in the entertainment/television field for 39 years (starting as a page, and concluding his career as a producer), he retired. He worked on such hits as "Truth or Consequences," "Queen For a Day," "It Could be You," "John F. Kennedy's 1960 Presidential Nomination," "The Steve Allen Show," "The Dean Martin Show," "Sanford and Son," "Too Close for Comfort," "What's Happening," "Carter Country," "Thicke of the Night," "The Jerry Lewis Talk Show," "Emmy Awards," and his last show, "Small Wonder." The list is long and impressive; therefore, it was not an easy adjustment to face.

Like a cruel slap in the face, this forced retirement was a harsh reality that needed acceptance. Norm braved the storm as a real

---

[33] See also Morris, et al. in the Bibliography.

trooper, a true hero, appearing to adjust immediately. When his last show was over, he knew his time had come to move aside for the younger crowd who would now drive Porsches, as we had done.

an evening with virginia satir

During this time, waiting for our house to sell, I had several interesting, valuable, and educational experiences happen.

One was a birthday gift from Diane, my graduate school friend. She took me to a premiere gala, Virginia Satir celebration, in the hills of Glendale. Virginia Satir, I learned from my graduate family-systems study, was a master therapist/educator. She invented a therapeutic theory and style called "People Sculpting," an innovative, revolutionizing technique which has since become universally renowned. I have a video cassette of this event sporting an intervention that she did on Claw. She explained the value of talking to various parts of the body - the injured parts especially. "Giving them love, by talking to them," is a healthy habit to have, she emphasized. This was not unlike the messages I gave my body, instinctively, following mother's death, when the little voice spoke in caressing, soothing tones to comfort me. I apply this technique today, as I falter sometimes in my daily routine.

The research shows that Transactional Analysis is used in Stroke Rehabilitation.

Oftentimes, the stroke patient will be faced with inner messages and experiences that are positive and supportive, like: "Don't be afraid, you have gone through the worst. You're alive and well, that's the main thing. You are still beautiful, even though you are not completely like before (pp. 51, 52).[34]

This quotation demonstrates the reparenting exercises similar to the inner messages I instinctively programmed.

I felt also blessed to copy for Diane the Virginia Satir videotape conferences, as a last video/editing project in my booth upstairs in my home. Viewing these tapes gave me added insight which Virginia hinted on at her celebration: I learned how to be gentle with my little child inside, loving her for the beautiful person she innately is — at all times. Perfect in all ways.

farewell to the old

Before we put our home up for sale, we tidied it up the best we could without a major redecorating overhaul. Norm hired Barbi Crosby, the spouse of his former high school chum Jack, as she was an aspiring interior decorator and we liked her interior design style. Barbi came up with some valued ideas. However, at one point, I told her in my newly expressive, direct stroke, uncool way, that I didn't like a particular idea she had. I did not mean to be rude, even though Norm told me of other incidents in restaurants, as an example, when my mouth sounded much like my mother's brazen style. Whatever I said, in whatever direct way, caused Barbi to burst into tears. I was ashamed at my insensitive, tactless remark, and apologized. I tried explaining this was a result of my right-hemisphere stroke head injury, for it did not

---

[34] See Champeau in the Bibliography.

sound like the usual, passive, quiet-as-a-mouse Marty.

"Patients exhibit a behavioral syndrome characterized as euphoric, tactless, irritable, lacking judgment, impulsive, and outspoken in a study of behavior change following rupture of anterior cerebral artery aneurysms."[35] My post-stroke personality alterations caused Barbi to feel so troubled at this incident, she phoned the American Heart/Stroke Council and requested literature on strokes; for she didn't understand this new person. I thought this was a very smart idea on her part.

During the selling of our home — which took 14 months and two realtors before the sale was consummated — our first realtor, Anita, took Norm and me to her fine Mulholland Country Club for a Sunday bunch. We ate a buffet that had every assortment of foods. It was a true feast, and I left replete. That evening, not wanting a heavy meal for dinner, Norm and I went to a local Mexican restaurant for a simple light meal. During the meal, I felt a pulling in my back area, way deep inside my body, an abnormal sensation that confused me. It was unusual, a feeling I had not had before. When I got home there was severe, unrelenting pain in my right side that I knew was unmistakably abnormal. I tried to steady myself, hoping it would go away. It increased in intensity. At 2:00 a.m., I insisted Norm drive me to the emergency hospital. I waited in line, for there were other people ahead of me in the emergency room.

Finally, the pain was so radical I lay down on the floor, as sitting was impossible. Norm spoke harshly to the personnel behind the counter, who were fixing their dinner in a microwave, telling them there was a severe emergency lying on their lobby floor.

---

[35] See Beckson and Cummings in the Bibliography.

They ushered me behind the curtains, insisting I have an EKG. "I'm not having a heart attack," I insisted, and one person asked, "How do you know you're not?" I admitted that he was right, and found myself wired up to their EKG machine. Later, confirmation proved I had not had a heart attack; rather, they suspected the cause to be a gallbladder attack. They gave me two injections of morphine, which did nothing.

I spent the night in the hospital. The next day, they took me upstairs for an ultrasound test, which revealed I had a severe gallbladder case, with stones in the main bile duct. I was fortunate to have the best emergency doctor in the hospital — the same hospital used for my angiogram.

Dr. Gittleman was quick to surmise the situation; he was ethical, gentle, and professional. I couldn't have been more fortunate. Lying in a bed, I recalled the familiar feeling I had while having my angiogram and bypass surgery. Dr. Sethi's name came to my mind. No sooner had I thought of him than I heard a familiar voice outside in the corridor. It was Dr. Sethi — in person! Another synchronicity, I thought. "Please tell Dr. Gittleman not to give me another stroke," I pleaded with my doctor friend. He made arrangements to speak with Dr. Gittleman, telling him about my case.

My gallbladder removal went well as expected, since they were unable to use the simple surgery because of the stones in the main bile duct. I had to have the full, traditional surgery, creating a scar that goes from under my left breast to the abdomen. There are so many scars on my body, I could play the role as a Frankenstein stand-in. Nevertheless, scars are what makes a person interesting, I feel. It adds character to an otherwise boring body — at least that's my rationalization now. An artist would appreciate me as a model for a medical diagram.

After this surgery, I felt finished with all the negative energies in my physical body. What could come next? I felt healthy, except for the occasional right hand numbing still plaguing me in the early mornings.

Shirley was the second realtor — who sold our house. Coincidentally, she went to high school with Norm and his friend, Jack Crosby. Shirley and I had also been friends in my early days in the Beverly Glen area, when I was married to my lawyer spouse. Shirley is sweet; focuses on eye contact when speaking to one and seemed to be a dedicated worker in our behalf. She and her partner (another Diane) sold our home in 14 weeks to a young couple who worked in the entertainment industry. Scott is a voice-over announcer, with a well-trained voice that one can easily discern currently heard on certain commercials. His spouse was in advertising promotions. Her name happened to be Martha Jane — the same as mine. I had never met, nor heard of, another person in my life who had the same name as I did. I still abhor my original name, regardless of another person sharing it.

Apparently, they loved our house instantly. The large cozy paneled den upstairs was perfect for Martha Jane's office, since she worked at home, and the audio/video booth was ideal for Scott's work. The downstairs also suited their lifestyle; for they had a six-month-old daughter, Meagan. However, I was not prepared for the future tragedy that this family endured. Their sad story will be revealed in time.

networking

With my mother gone, and having sold our house, I was able to make a move to Leisure World by myself, to check it out, seeing whether it was everything we had dreamed and hoped for. I was fearful, however, leaving my dear Norm, wondering if I could really make it by myself with only one functioning hand. We decided I'd rent an apartment first, so I could investigate the potential.

Another synchronicity surfaced earlier, adding to this decision. Norm worked with a casting director on his shows, named David, who seemed to know everyone; his networking abilities were incredible. David also attended the Science-of-Mind Church and was responsible for originally connecting us with Domenic Polifrone, the inspiring minister of the Hollywood Church of Religious Science, where I took my practitioner classes.

One day David, Norm, and I had lunch together in a Greek restaurant on Ventura Boulevard in Sherman Oaks. While chatting about our anticipated move, I innocently mentioned that I wished I knew someone in Leisure World, whom I could talk to before we made this move. David immediately said, "I do — I know someone who lives there, and her name is Sally." He went on to say she was a beautiful person whom he knew while in England. David put us in contact with Sally. She willingly showed us her condominium in Leisure World, which Norm and I connected with immediately, due to the abundance of light it offered, as well as the loft design. I also related well with Sally, for she was a young, talented business person. She is on the art counsel at the Los Angeles County Museum, and had organized other newly formed art museums, art galleries; albeit widowed at a young age. Sally introduced us to June, her realtor. June located my new apartment and later found our designer home.

greeting new challenges

This introduction to Sally gave me a feeling of security, and I was ready and eager to sever my bonds with my Studio City neighborhood, knowing I would see Norm on the weekends, and this would be a test to my burgeoning independence.

Before I left, I prepared myself for this move into the unknown Orange County area — a distance from the Studio City area — by taking a "Safe Driver" test at Northridge Hospital. I had to drive alone before they could appraise my driving abilities. The neurologist at the hospital cast doubt about my ever driving again, which frightened me. I wanted clarification of my capacity to drive from professionals.

Two persons took me out on the road for the first time. I was in a strange car that was equipped with two steering wheels. It had a unique, different design for the turn indicators; the entire construction was for the disabled in every situation. This was the first time I had driven in six years. I was in a foreign car, in a polluted area, with high traffic, at the peak hour — if there is such a thing in Los Angeles — and on unfamiliar streets. "Drive," they commanded. "Turn here." "Turn there." "Back up there." "Go right there." "Now turn left at the first busy intersection; go two blocks, make a right and then swing a U. Now head for the freeway entrance."

"Freeway?" I exclaimed. Oh my, I thought. Please God, help me. The two persons did not see my knees shaking, nor feel my right palm sweating. I hope it doesn't slip on the steering wheel, I thought during this command.

My prayers saved the day. I did a splendid job; and they both congratulated me, saying, "Why haven't you driven before this?"

they asked in a genuine tone. Whew! I thought, wiping my brow and hand on my clothes. I passed my greatest fear. I drove! I actually drove — and on the freeway! It was a "yippee" feeling that was like a deep down, bubble-up, surging experience, exploding rapidly into my system and soul.

I packed up a small amount of my clothes, some cosmetics and insignificant items myself, putting things into boxes friends helped collect. Mentally, I considered myself ready to leave. My new apartment had decor in a pastel Southwestern theme. The apartment, including rented furniture, had all the amenities and utilities. I had a tiny view of the city lights that flickered outside the dining room window. It had a small balcony with padded redwood lawn furniture. I sat out there daily, for the outdoors was a pleasant interlude.

During the week I was a glutton for activities. I read the Leisure World News, selecting the most exciting clubs and lectures to attend. The menu was immense. My calendar bulged from so many choices. I went to the Parapsychology Club, to hear lectures on the occult and mystical magic. At the Walt Whitman Circle, they read *Leaves of Grass*, in between discussions. There were meetings on current events and community interests, such as: travel films, movies, plays; everything, even a video club! I took many classes from A-to-Z offered by the emeritus program of Saddleback College. In finances, I was inept; but in writing, I excelled. Under the tutelage of Elizabeth, I completed my autobiography; and from MJ, a talented young screenwriter, I was encouraged to continue writing nonfiction. Each assignment was read aloud before the class, from whom I learned.

I perused the bus system routes and was able to transport myself in and around Laguna Hills, making friends; many friends! The first were Flo and Al, who is aphasic. I met Al while on a walk in my neighborhood. He had fallen on the sidewalk. I picked him up like the proud street-walker that I was. Even though he couldn't talk, Al's eyes said "Thank you." We communicated nonverbally. Flo, his devoted spouse, became my good friend, needing me as her "chatterbox therapist." It isn't easy being the caregiver of a stroke person. Ask Norm.

Other friends, like flowers, became my fragrant role models. Among them were Betty and Arthur, both expressive published poets; D-Dancer — a line dancer at 80-something! Ida, my devoted dissertation editor (Thanks, Ida!); and Connie, who gave meditation sessions in her condominium; Frieda, a Scrabble nut; Mike, my golfer neighbor; and petite Dottie showed me the public transportation. For 15 cents we rode to the elegant Newport/Fashion Island outdoor mall. I thought I had arrived in paradise. It sounds like a Who's Who list — but more preferred.

I walked everywhere at first, but later Norm bought me a blue golf cart, with fringe, that buzzed me around the area in grand style. I was even able to travel in a tunnel, under the crowded street, where I ended up on the other side, at the mall in my neighborhood. It was heaven on wheels.

On the weekends, Norm joined me, bringing more of my clothes; his car was splitting at the seams from so much collected belongings. While with me, he'd market and prepare delicious meals which I could eat during his time at the Studio City house during the week. The escrow was about to close.

When the enormous, overwhelming job of packing a 3400-square-foot house was finished - thanks to Norm's daughter, J'me, who appeared after work, and my daughter, Jeni, giving furniture away to children, causes, friends, and neighbors — it was time to wave good-bye to 15 years of living in the same house.

Norm moved into my small, two-bedroom apartment with me. We put all the furniture and hundreds of boxes into the empty garage of our new home in Leisure World, which soon was to become a designer quality showcase home. Norm hired our former neighbor Joanna to decorate it. She was from the early Studio City neighborhood where our cantilevered home was, on Sunshine Terrace. He called it his bachelor pad. This was where he courted me. Joanna had moved to Laguna Beach, to live among the other artists in the colony, noted for its artistic freedom. Her move was another synchronicity: she was within minutes of our home, and therefore convenient for her decorating creativity.

At this point in time we are still nested here, enjoying Joanna's choice of teal and raspberry colors (still my favorite), and with a double front entrance door in leaded glass and crystal that creates dancing rainbow reflections on the purple rug in the hallway, from the filtered light through the curved designs. It is an *Architectural Digest* wonder.

During our apartment stay, Joanna was busy putting this outstanding creation together. One evening we received a call from Scott, the new owner of our former Studio City home. He called and said he had awful news to report, but we were to call back in 15 minutes. He also stated, "But don't ask for Martha Jane, if someone strange picks up the receiver."

This was odd, we thought. We wondered whether something was wrong with the house. Norm called back, as instructed, on the speakerphone, so we both could listen.

Scott answered, his trained, mellow voice quivering. "Martha Jane died," he blurted, bluntly.

Died? We couldn't believe his words. No, this was too unreal.

It wasn't true. They had only been there 16 days. She was only 28 years old.

"Yes, it's true," he said. "She was in the kitchen about to prepare me a meal, when I came home early. While she opened her mouth to tell me that the contractors were coming Wednesday, she keeled over, in the middle of her sentence, dead before she hit the yellow kitchen floor. She had an instant heart attack," he cried in agony.

My God. We both felt horrid. I had never met them, having been living in Laguna Hills, but I did speak with Martha Jane over the phone once, and we had discussed our same names, so I felt a natural kinship connection with her. Apparently, she ceased taking her heart medication because she had been breast-feeding and didn't want her young daughter, Meagan, contaminated by the medicine. Both Scott and her doctor did not know she had stopped the medication, nor did they know the severity of her weak heart condition.

It was a tragedy difficult to dismiss. I grieved for months, even though I did not know them intimately; I felt I did, and that we were personal friends, or family. It reminded me that life is so infinitely fragile, so short, so delicate, that each instant is for living, getting your hands dirty with everyday grime, with a spirit that includes every reasonable risk one can invent, or realize.

Chapter 14

KNOWLEDGE ILLUMINATES THE PATH

debris, diagnoses, discoveries

MANY SYNCHRONICITIES STARTLED MY CONSCIOUSNESS, BEGGING ME TO BE A believer by now. The student was ready. Synchronicities followed a significant stream along my path of becoming whole. The first to initiate the flow was a phone call from Susan, my former hospital roommate. She related how she was considering having a pioneering procedure to help stimulate blood flow to her injured spinal cord. A Boston doctor conducted it. He took blood vessels from the intestine area, implanting them either in the brain for a stroke victim, or into the spinal cord in her case. It piqued my interest, for she said it was on its way to becoming scientifically proven, although in the early stages: it was intended to help stroke persons recover from their aphasia or perception handicaps! It sounded like a miracle; however, it was expensive, as well as experimental.

I wanted to speak with this doctor, as Susan said he was visiting in my Orange County area. I placed a phone call to this inventive doctor; at first, reaching his answering service. He returned my call within minutes, detailing the general concept of his procedure, querying me on my condition as well. I explained my complicated medical history. After interviewing each other over a half hour by phone, he determined I was too far along in my healing process, and his new medical design would not benefit me. He did recommend, however, that I see a well-established, competent neurologist in the Newport Beach area named Dr. O'Carroll, who could offer help with my still numb right hand. I made the appointment for the following week. My numbness was becoming painful by now, and that hand was most vital for my survival.

As I walked into Dr. O'Carroll's office, immediately I liked the vibrations, as well as his quiet, professional demeanor. When it came time to explain my numbness, I said: "Perhaps, in my non-professional diagnosis, it is Carpel Tunnel Syndrome."

He said, "Let's see," and escorted me to an examining room where he tested the hand with electrical devices, showing squiggly lines and colors on a monitor. "Congratulations on your diagnosis," he said, promptly. "You have an advanced case of Carpel Tunnel Syndrome. If it isn't taken care of very soon, you may lose the use of your thumb completely." Oh my God, I thought. Here I go again, with flashbacks of Dr. King's office so long ago.

Dr. O'Carroll gave me the name of a hand surgeon, Dr. Cook who directed me to the best alternatives. I was moving along rapidly on the next phase of my path. Before I continue detailing my path further, there is one final footnote to finish this section completely.

One night Norm and I tuned into "20/20," ABC's weekly

program. We found it interesting to see the Boston doctor on one of their segments describing his new theory and method. It was not a glowing report, for the inference was quackery. I'm thankful I did not delve into it further, and thus was glad the synchronicities led me to the other doctors; so the negative debris became eliminated from my path entirely.

Dr. O'Carroll's referral, Dr. Cook, explained two methods of correcting this Carpal Tunnel Syndrome. One, which he recommended, was to cut the palm lengthwise, correcting the condition; but, this method would prevent me from using my hand for about six months. How could I do this, I wondered. It was the only functioning hand I had. Another alternative was to enter the palm with a thin, paper-cut-like incision, executing the surgery like an endoscopy. This made more practical sense, although Dr. Cook did not recommend this, as he had not performed this surgery more than a few times. It was a new technique. He had a colleague who did this, however, and referred me to him.

Dr. Hammitt had an entire medical center, adjacent to a hospital, where he performed this type of laser hand surgery, with a high success rate. I had this new surgery done on one July morning, and was able to use my right hand that same night, without pain, without problems. It was another miracle in motion. The only remaining evidence of this surgery is a one-eighth-inch fine line in the middle of my right palm that blends with all my other palm wrinkles. I asked Dr. Hammitt what causes Carpal Tunnel Syndrome problems. He said, "A hormonal change." That made sense, for when I reviewed the time the numbness began, my hormones were uncontrolled, like an untamed beast. The numbness seemed not connected to my right eye blackness. They were two separate conditions.

To think all these years not one doctor came up with this diagnosis is disgusting, and sad. I have not had another numb feeling since that surgery terminated, several years ago. I presume I needed to get all the boulders out of my path before I could continue on my journey.

Along with attending the stroke Support Club meetings in Leisure World, which were similar to the meetings in my old area — just different faces, different speakers, different format — I also took another new risk. I saw in the Leisure World News an advertisement for Transcendental Meditation: "Free Introductory Offer," the advertisement read. I became interested in this technique; however, it was off the campus, located about 2 miles from my home area. Ready for another challenge, I decided to satisfy my curiosity, and called Dial-A-Ride, a public transportation bus that picks up people who phone in advance. It only costs a dollar.

I made contact with this transportation, and was delivered to a wellness institute in a medical center. I waited in a small empty room, circled with fabric chairs. I waited for someone to greet me, to explain the details. During the wait I glanced at the leaflets, brochures, and books that casually lay scattered in the single dark bookshelf. The literature appealed to me. Soon a tall, slender, poised, middle-aged, dark-haired person, in a white laboratory coat, entered with stethoscopes poking from his pocket. Oh, not another doctor, I thought. He introduced himself as Dr. Michael Grossman, a family practitioner. He explained the significance of Transcendental Meditation, the focus of the course; and the price, since he was the instructor. He asked about my condition. I readily disclosed my history. He inquired if I were interested in attending weekly group sessions on Attitudinal Healing at this center.

I realized this was the information I had seen and read while waiting for him. I knew Attitudinal Healing was originated by Dr. Jerry Jampolsky, in Tiburon in Northern California. I had read most of his appealing books on healing, taken from *The Course in Miracles*, now nationally known in centers throughout the country. I felt delighted by this invitation and told him I would love to come to a support group, but I would need a ride, explaining my non-driving condition. He was certain someone in the Leisure World area could drive me. He said he'd post my name on the bulletin board. I wasn't that positive it would develop, thinking it was similar to an engagement promise; but if it did manifest, I would eagerly accept. Two weeks later, a person phoned me, volunteering to pick me up. I felt thrilled, for I had made another attempt at healing myself. That was four years ago. I am still going, and have become a co-facilitator, and sometimes facilitator, in this group, when my school classes permit. The group stimulates my mind, and touches my heart, for each meeting is different, with a message of love that generally connects us with absolute, unconditional love. It is enlightening. It is pure beauty.

Dr. Grossman became my primary general physician in my new area. One office visit he checked my body, noticing that my left leg, otherwise named Stump, appeared diminished in circulation. "Oh no," I moaned again, perhaps louder than usual. Another medical challenge, I questioned. An ultrasound commenced, finding a 75 percent blockage in my left leg. It was nothing to write home about; for I directly saw a vascular surgeon in the area who told me to refrain from being anxiously concerned — at this time. He also assured me that my Takayasus Disease was probably gone — if indeed I really had it — stating that its symptoms generally appear like a billowing surge or terrible tornado. It does its havoc, then vanishes as quickly as it comes, similar to the flu, he analyzed with his analogy.

That was terrific news. I could write home about that! I speculated that this was the reason my left leg usually felt like an amputee's stump. How should anyone know, unless they have a paralyzed leg, or a leg amputated, I pondered.

Shortly after this miracle, my son Randy, a commercial realtor in the Irvine area, spoke casually about his clients, a new graduate school, located in the Irvine area. Simultaneously my inner voice told me it was time to go back to graduate school, finishing what I had started seven years earlier but hadn't completed! I shared this dream with Randy. Another synchronicity was poking me again.

Immediately, I phoned and made an appointment with Pat, the attractive raven-haired director of the school. Later I met Dr. Bonnie Price, the well-organized, creative, businessperson, president of Western American University. I thought I could benefit from this school, for it offered not only an M.A. degree in Psychology but also a Ph.D. in Psychology, which later was changed to a Psychology Doctorate (Psy.D.) degree, since the university was a neophyte and needed more research provisions to qualify for Ph.D. candidates. Nevertheless, it suited my intentions and needs, for a Doctor of Psychology was more clinically useful for my mission — as Dr. Backarack (Psy.D.) had demonstrated years ago. I signed up immediately and began taking classes the following September. To top it off, I began driving myself to classes (a pleasing feat unto myself) but at this point still avoiding the freeways: a leftover phobia from the Northridge Hospital's neurologist and his foreboding; but I have a direct shot to the school on the highways. Moreover, I am ready to work on my freeway phobia now.

Class by class continued, according to its long list of state requirements, and my enthusiasm followed each one, now having received 15 "credit with honors" — according to their non-grading system. I am unable to say which class stimulated more interest, for I read every book in the field as a hobby. Textbooks are my reading pleasure; therefore, the subjects challenged my interest, naturally.

The final photo in the photograph section depicts me standing on the next-to-the-last step, holding up my M.A. diploma. This photo was a surprise, and a shock to see, for rarely have I seen Claw in a photograph — all tightly clenched. It was an embarrassing feeling to view it in this light, wishing that he, or she, was normal. At the same time, my pride overshadowed the embarrassment. Norm calls Claw my badge of honor; so I will treat it with respect and allow Claw to gracefully become my teacher, achieving my dreams, and wrestling all other hurdles with me, as in the past, on this journey. The work ahead is evident, for me as well as for Norm.

work

It needs to be said that "strokes not only affect the patient's employment but also that of the individuals who find themselves primarily responsible for the patient's care. Return to work offers a useful measure of economic independence but is a relatively crude index of recovery. It is dependent upon the age of the patient, the economic resources available, the type of work, the occupational status held and whether the work can be altered to suit the patient."[36]

---

[36] See Newman in the Bibliography for a complete citation.

miscellaneous findings, facts and notes

This section attempts to convey various facts and findings that are equally significant, yet do not fit into a specific part of my narrative, some of which may seem surprising. For instance, in older patients, strokes occur more frequently at rest; in younger ones, more frequently during activity. Hypertension was least common in the oldest group. A history of transient ischemic attacks was significantly related to a good outcome. Patients who sustained their stroke during activity are more likely to have a good outcome. Brain stem lesions are not visualized on CT scans. Motivation and mood state are assessed by therapists and psychologists, respectively, and proved highly significant predictors of outcome. The majority of stroke patients are over 65 years of age.

The great fear is having a second stroke. Some localized brain lesions are correlated with specific intellectual dysfunction, but two patients with the same lesion will often suffer different defects. Some patients' problems are unfortunately overlooked, because the patients appear to understand (or don't physically look different). Therefore, an accurate assessment of comprehension is necessary before intervention can be planned.[37]

Recovery is equally likely to occur at any stage due to behavioral strategy changes. One should focus on health-orientated treatment, rather than illness. Primary social work interest and involvement have been with patients' families.

Literature readings for the interested reader include a humorous approach by Sacks, *The Man Who Mistook his Wife for a Hat and Other Clinical Tales*, which offers comical wisdom, educating and

---

[37] See Evans and Miller in the Bibliography.

enlightening a serious subject with amusement. Equally entertaining in addition, along a related vein, one can find personal essays about neuropsychological patients. Offering clinical data is in Klawans' Newton's Madness: Further Tales of Clinical Neurology. The most valuable reference manual I found is Pinel, my reliable and trusted source.

However, the most comforting narrative edition for recovering stroke patients, is by Veith, Can You Hear the Clapping of One Hand? Within this volume I felt her presence, and pain, as mine. She refreshed my mind of a diminished tactile sensibility that interferes with my ability to feel the results of a runny nose. The term is called hypesthesia. I was unaware of this term, but cognizant of the condition. She also taught me that when walking up stairs the unimpaired foot goes first, whereas in walking downstairs the injured leg proceeds. I usually do not go up stairs unless there is a banister on my right side. She also spoke about her husband using soft-spoken words or a gesture to remind her when she has food on the left side of her face, unable to feel it. Norm and I have a code, although at times he looks like a lost lizard looking for water — his tongue frantically darting in and out of his mouth — yet unobtrusively trying to hide his signal from casual outsiders. Recently I found a small oval mirror that fits on a finger that aids in discovering food on my face by myself. Signals like these are important strategies the rehabilitation therapists sometimes try to use in their retraining programs.

The author Veith and I shared getting lost in unfamiliar places — if we are not careful to note landmarks. I am especially vulnerable in complicated malls. Also, both of us acknowledged the distressing sensation if our mate/caregiver is ill. We feel defenseless if something happens to them, abandoned, frightened, and helpless.

We both felt our spouse must have knowledge of physical therapy. And we confessed our strange condition called "foot drop," which means our left shoe does not always stay securely placed on the foot. Occasionally, I have found my shoe somewhere along my path, as I am unable to feel my foot, mentioned earlier.

Strokes are devastating. The reality demands change, adaptation to one's basic structure. Thus, knowledge surrounding the physiology is necessary to impart.

Therefore, knowing that knowledge illuminates the path, I will offer more stroke facts, taken from the American Heart Stroke Association, shedding additional light for others on this devastating condition.

Before commencing I will remark, as an interesting aside, that one day sitting in our car in a gas station, I waited as Norm filled our tank. I heard a commentary on the radio that said, in essence: researchers have found that women of menopausal ages can acquire strange blood disorders, affecting their health. Because of my condition my ears perked up. I cannot offer scientific evidence regarding that statement. However, during my research, I found the title, "Relationship of menopause to cardiovascular disease,"[38] which I thought would solve this mystery. It did not link to any library location, unfortunately.

However, as mentioned, the information that deserves most notice is a simplified version of what I have been striving to express in this narrative. There is some repetitive overlap from the earlier sections. I feel justified, for much of it is worded differently, with new material inserted. One needs to be informed thoroughly with all realities in the serious matter of possibly saving lives. Following

---

[38] See Kuller in the Bibliography.

that, an insert on my own "helpful hints," taken from my personal experiences, unfolds, as well as subjective feelings about the importance of a supportive spouse, friends and further education. My speculations concerning this retroflective process will also stimulate commentary. After this section, the conclusion, stated in the final chapter *Light Beyond the Rainbow* summarizes, with implications, themes, generalizations, and questions for future investigators, thus completing the dissertation in this final process of my journey. The epilogue, stating Bowlby's Attachment and Loss Theory, follows; accompanied with grief therapy solutions, and suggestions, concluding the document. A glossary is appended.

discovery: stroke facts and information

Thus, the most helpful education, presenting the current facts, as The American Heart Association states:

What Is a Stroke?

A stroke occurs when a blood vessel bringing oxygen and nutrients to part of the brain bursts or becomes clogged. When that happens the nerve cells in that part of the brain can't function.

The nerve cells of the brain control how we receive and interpret sensations. They also control most of our bodily movements.

When some nerve cells in the brain can't function, then the part of the body controlled by them can't function either. This can result in difficulty speaking, the inability to walk, or loss of memory, among other symptoms.

The effects of a stroke may be very slight or severe, temporary or permanent. It depends in part on which brain cells have been damaged, how widespread the damage is, how well the body repairs the blood supply system to the brain, or how quickly other areas of brain tissue take over the work of the damaged cells.

What a person is like before a stroke also determines to some degree how he or she will react afterward, although stroke can mask or magnify personality traits. One person may struggle to overcome her handicap, while another becomes resigned, requiring much encouragement from his family and others.

Recovering from a stroke depends on the amount and location of brain damage, the person's general health, his or her personality and emotional state, the support of friends and loved ones, and the care the person receives.

The Blood Supply to the Brain

To function, brain cells must have a continuous, ample supply of oxygen and other nutrients from the blood. If brain cells are completely deprived of blood for more than a short period of time, they die. It follows that the blood supply system to the brain is very important.

How does this blood supply system work? The blood is pumped from the heart to the brain through a network of blood vessels-elastic tubes called arteries. The arteries in the brain are called cerebral arteries. They branch into smaller arteries and finally into tiny, thin-walled vessels called capillaries. It's through the capillaries that the nutrients in blood reach each of the millions of minute nerve cells in brain tissue. Interference or damage in this supply system causes stroke.

How Strokes Occur

The blood supply of the brain may be disrupted by different events. Sometimes it's hard to determine the cause or causes of a particular stroke, so a doctor may need time to make a definite diagnosis.

One of the most common causes of stroke is the blocking of a cerebral artery by a clot, called thrombus, that forms inside the artery. This is called cerebral thrombosis. Sometimes the clot occurs in one of four neck arteries that normally transport oxygen-rich blood from the heart to the brain.

A clot isn't likely to occur in a healthy artery. But sometimes arteries are damaged by atherosclerosis, an abnormal condition in which a thick, rough deposit forms on their inner wall and gradually narrows the passageway so the blood flow slows. The roughened deposits build up and jut into the bloodstream. When that happens, blood is likely to clot around the projections.

Sometimes a wandering blood clot, called an embolus, is carried in the bloodstream. It may be a piece of a larger clot from a neck vessel or from a heart damaged by disease. If the clot gets stuck in one of the cerebral arteries, a process called cerebral embolism will interfere with blood flow to the brain.

Stroke can also occur when a diseased artery in the brain bursts and floods the surrounding delicate tissue with blood. This is called a cerebral hemorrhage. The cells nourished by the artery don't get their supply of food and oxygen and can't do their job. Also, the accumulation of blood from the ruptured artery soon clots, which displaces brain tissue and interferes with brain function. This causes mild-to-severe symptoms. Cerebral hemorrhages are more likely to occur in people who suffer from a combination of atherosclerosis and high blood pressure.

Cerebral hemorrhages also may be caused by a head injury or when an aneurysm bursts. Aneurysms are blood-filled pouches that balloon out from a weak spot in the artery wall. The weakness in the artery wall is present at birth, but the aneurysm doesn't usually develop until adult life. Often it's associated with high blood pressure. Aneurysms don't always cause serious trouble, but when they burst, the result is a stroke.

How the Supply System Repairs Itself

Whenever the blood supply is cut off from an area, a

remarkable thing happens. The body attempts a repair job. Small neighboring arteries get larger and take over part of the damaged artery's work. In this way nerve cells temporarily put out of order may recover, although other cells, still lacking an adequate blood supply, die. If the blood supply is cut off by a clot, there are mechanisms in the blood that may dissolve the clot.

When damaged cells recover, the part of the body they control may eventually improve or even return to normal. A paralyzed muscle may recover its strength; lost speech may return; impaired memory may be restored.

When a stroke is caused by a clot or embolus in a very small artery, the outlook for recovery is usually better than when an artery bursts.

Stroke Risk Factors

Regular medical check-ups are the best protection against stroke. By taking a medical history and making an examination, a doctor can detect the risk factors that predispose a person to stroke. The preventive treatment can begin at an early age, when it's more effective.

Some risk factors can be treated; others can't. The factors that can be treated are:

High Blood Pressure - Hypertension is the most important risk factor for stroke. In fact, stroke risk varies directly with blood pressure. If high blood pressure is controlled, the risk of stroke is greatly reduced. That's why everyone's blood pressure should be checked regularly. Often blood pressure can be controlled simply by eating a healthier diet and maintaining proper weight. Drugs to control blood pressure are also available.

Heart Disease - Independent of blood pressure, people with heart problems have more than twice the risk of stroke than people with normal hearts. Anyone with any type of heart disease should see a doctor regularly. Good management of heart disease reduces the risk of stroke.

Cigarette Smoking - Recent studies show that cigarette smoking is an important risk factor for stroke. Stopping reduces the risk of stroke, even in long-time smokers.

High Red Blood Count - An increase in the red blood count is a risk factor for stroke. The reason is that increased red blood cells thicken the blood and make clots more likely. This problem is treatable by removing blood or administering "blood thinners." A complete blood count (CBC) is a simple test that can detect this problem. It's usually part of a routine physical examination.

Transient Ischemic Attacks (TIAs) - Only about 10 percent of strokes are preceded by mini-strokes. Nevertheless, TIAs are extremely important; they're strong predictors of stroke. TIAs are usually treated with drugs that inhibit clots from forming.

The risk factors that can't be changed are:

Age - Older people have a much greater stroke risk than younger people.

Being Male - Men have a greater risk of stroke than women.

Race - African-Americans have much greater risk of death and disability from stroke than whites. This may be because African-Americans are more likely to have high blood pressure.

Diabetes Mellitus - Although diabetes is treatable, having it makes a person much more likely to suffer a stroke. This is even more true for women than for men. Many times, diabetics also have high blood pressure, increasing their risk of stroke even more.

Prior Stroke - The risk of stroke for someone who's already had one is many times that of someone who has not. *Heredity* - Stroke risk is greater for people who have a family history of stroke.

Besides the risk factors listed, other (controllable) factors indirectly increase stroke risk. These include: 1) elevated blood cholesterol and lipids, 2) excessive alcohol intake, 3) physical inactivity and 4) obesity.

These are secondary risk factors. They affect the risk of

stroke indirectly by increasing the risk of heart disease (which is a primary risk factor for stroke).

Some rather low-level risk factors — when combined with other risk factors — become very important. Taking oral contraceptives and smoking cigarettes, for example, increases the risk of stroke considerably. More to the point, the 10 percent of the population in whom one-third of all strokes occur have a set of five risk factors. These are: 1) high blood pressure, 2) elevated blood cholesterol levels, 3) abnormal glucose tolerance, 4) cigarette smoking and 5) left ventricular hypertrophy (the over-development of the left side of the heart). People who have all these factors should have close medical supervision.

Stroke Warning Signs

Often doctors can detect signs and symptoms that may mean a stroke is about to occur. In fact, your own body may warn you of an impending stroke. It does this by certain symptoms you can recognize and tell your doctor about. These symptoms are:

1. A sudden weakness or numbness of the face, arm, leg on one side of the body.
2. Sudden dimness or loss of vision, particularly in one eye.
3. Loss of speech, or trouble talking or understanding speech.
4. Sudden severe headaches with no apparent cause.

5. Unexplained dizziness, unsteadiness or sudden falls, especially along with any of the previous symptoms.

Treatment

If a doctor finds that these signs or symptoms are caused by a blocked artery leading to the brain, surgery may be performed to remove the block and reduce the risk of stroke. This type of surgery is sometimes used to try to prevent recurring strokes, too. Other techniques that surgeons use include removing blood clots and clipping off aneurysms to prevent re-bleeding.

Drugs that delay blood clotting (anticoagulants) may be prescribed for some people, both to avert a first stroke or prevent a second one. Always consult your doctor before taking any of these agents.

Although there's no rule about recurrence of strokes, someone who's had one has a very high risk of having another. Good general medical follow-up programs can help control stroke risk factors and reduce the risk of another stroke.

Once a stroke has occurred, the most important step in current treatment is developing a sound rehabilitation program.

Recovery and Rehabilitation

Some people are only slightly affected by a stroke. Others recover quickly from what seem like severe strokes. Still others may suffer such serious damage that it takes a long time for them to regain even partial use of their limbs, speech or whatever has been affected.

For many people who recover quickly and spontaneously, rehabilitation isn't a serious problem. But a doctor should be called at once when a person shows signs of a stroke. Then he or she can take measures to improve the chance of recovery. Much can be done to help some people who are partially paralyzed or whose speech has been affected by stroke. Even people seriously paralyzed by stroke may make remarkable progress toward becoming self-sufficient.

Three Keys to Successful Rehabilitation

For rehabilitation to be most effective, three points must be kept in mind:

1. Rehabilitation must begin as soon after the stroke as possible.
2. The family can be the affected person's most important source of support during rehabilitation.
3. Rehabilitation is a team effort with the doctor, nurse, and other specialists working with the person and family.

For a Stroke Patient's Family

Families should know how much the recovering person has been affected, and what lies ahead as a result of the stroke. The adjustment period may be hard for both patient and family, but understanding the person's condition and being prepared for it helps. Then realistic goals can be set.

Understanding Behavior

People who've had a stroke may have emotional upsets they can't control. They cry easily, laugh inappropriately, and may be irritated with little provocation. Usually these effects of stroke don't last very long. The important thing is for recovering people and their families to realize that these behavioral problems are due to the stroke and don't express the person's true feelings.

Periods of depression are common and natural, if they aren't too deep or prolonged. Because their progress is slow, people with stroke may become indifferent to relearning skills they once took for granted. Recovering people are also likely to be sensitive about their condition and may become suspicious of what people are thinking about them.

They need constant encouragement to overcome their depression and face up to their problems. If depression persists, tell the doctor. In some cases he or she may decide to prescribe medication to ease the depression.

Sometimes the judgment of people who've had a stroke is impaired; they may have memory lapses, too. In spite of these losses, they may be mentally alert and capable in other respects. Families shouldn't hesitate to have a frank talk with the doctor about the mental changes making them anxious.

Professional advice is especially needed at this time. Such guidance can help families resolve their own adjustment difficulties. The American Heart Association has informative booklets for families coping with behavioral changes following stroke.

Resolving the conflicts that an altered personality creates in a household isn't easy. But it can be accomplished with the patience, tact and understanding of all family members. Giving the recovering person something to live for is half the battle. Most people can learn to care for themselves and assume some household duties, even if they can't return to gainful employment. Families can also help recovering members develop new outside interests within their capacities.

Fortunately in many people the early effects of stroke disappear or remain to only a slight degree.

Helping Someone with a Speech Difficulty

When a stroke affects the speech centers of the brain, the

ability to use language is also affected. This condition is called aphasia. Aphasia takes various forms. For example, someone may be able to understand words but not be able to say or write them; or the ability to read or use numbers may be affected.

Despite these problems, it's important for families to realize that people with aphasia haven't necessarily lost the power to think clearly. They should be included in family decision-making, especially about issues involving them. Remember that they understand far more than they seem to; never say anything near someone with aphasia that you don't want him to her to know.

It's helpful to have speech difficulty evaluated by a professional speech therapist as soon as possible after the acute illness is over. Such an evaluation can be the basis for planning a speech retraining program.

Often a family member can conduct the program if a therapist isn't regularly available.

Studies have shown that people who've had a stroke make the most progress when speech retraining begins as soon as possible.

Self-Help Devices

A number of simple, practical self-help devices exist that enable handicapped people to become more self-reliant.

Also a doctor, physical and occupational therapists, or the visiting nurse service can give advice about possible household adjustments.

Often a handyman's skills may be just as useful as commercial gadgets. Here are a few ideas you may find useful.

1. Handrails can be fastened along walls for people who have trouble walking. They can be put up by anyone handy with tools, but be sure that they (or anything that will be grasped or relied on) are fastened securely.

2. A rubber mat for the floor of the shower stall or bottom of the tub makes bathing easier and safer.

3. Soap enclosed in a washcloth pouch isn't as likely to slip from the hands. A hand grasp on the wall is also a good idea.

4. If the recovering person is confined to a wheelchair, cut a plywood board to fit on the chair arms and around his or her waist. It can be used as a worktable for games, writing or meals.

5. Specially designed card holders, typewriters and telephones, as well as other helpful items, are useful for people who can only use one arm.

6. People who must spend a good deal of time in bed should have a bedside table with toilet articles within easy reach and a bell for summoning members of the household. A light switch should also be within reach.

7. Housewives who've been affected by a stroke can still carry on their work with the help of nonskid mixing bowls, lapboards and other such devices.

A member of the family can, with a little resourcefulness, solve many minor but troublesome problems. It may be necessary to get rid of small scatter rugs and unnecessary doorsills and to rearrange furniture and other hazards to walking in the home.

Whatever one can do to help the recovering person help himself is good medicine — physically and psychologically.

Suggestions for Long-Term Care

Here are suggestions for families of people who require long-term care:

1. Divide duties so the full burden of care doesn't fall on one family member.
2. Accept help from friends who volunteer. Friends often want to help but need a family member to tell them how they can be most helpful.
3. Help the recovering person take responsibility for exercising regularly.
4. Gradually and easily let the recovering person assume responsibility for self-care and other activities. This calls for fine judgment to encourage independence but not promote unrealistic expectations. If she can brush her teeth, comb her hair or dress herself, let her do so even if it takes a long time.
5. Praise any successful effort, and don't be discouraged by failures. Recovering from stroke is a slow process.
6. Have the recovering person participate in as much

family planning as he or she can. Feeling useful is a tremendous morale booster.

7. Help the recovering person stay in contact with the world. Don't push him to the sidelines and trust the television and radio to fill the time.

8. Encourage him to develop a hobby. Spend time together — perhaps playing chess, checkers, or bridge would be fun.

9. Encourage people to visit if the person's condition warrants it. Make the person feel wanted and a part of the social picture.

10. Check with the doctor regularly. And call if things aren't going the way you think they should.

The aforementioned information is important and useful. They are facts to acquaint oneself with.

If each stroke person wrote his or her personal narrative, there would be different stories, for each stroke is different, depending upon where the injury is located in the brain. On the other hand, there are so many similarities. It is a paradox: different, yet similar.[39] Right hemisphere injuries can result in using poor judgment, which is one reason the neurologist in Northridge Hospital gave me such a gloomy prediction for driving again. It is known that right hemisphere strokees *think* they can drive, where in reality, their judgment can be severely impaired, resulting in risky behavior on the road. Conversely, generally left hemisphere impairment does not result in as dangerous a risk, compared with the right hemisphere's driving

---

[39] See Shemel'kov in the Bibliography.

capability. It does depend on the severity of injury as to a driving prognosis.

my personal helpful hints

I have other helpful hints and suggestions from my personal experience. A few are:

1. Have someone sew elastic thread, expanding it, on buttons with long sleeved blouses and shirts, so the hands can slip in easily.

2. Get from the beauty supply, a washable, mesh, zippered "hood" that can be worn over the head while dressing, so make-up cannot soil clothes.

3. Find from the hospital occupational services, or handicap medical supply, a curved, rocker-type knife for cutting meat and vegetables.

4. Women, if you have only the use of one hand, learn to wear elastic midi-length skirts, with colorful knee-length flat boots or sandals in the summer. I've found boots are much easier to pull up with one hand. (I'm having difficulty finding Velcro tennis shoes in stores. However, recently I located elastic shoelaces in a nearby mall, making tennis shoes less of a problem.)

5. Women, splurge and find a friendly salon that has a waxing technician — if you can afford it — and treat yourself occasionally to a leg waxing, and eyebrow arch and tint. (Once I got "pluck happy" with my "left-side neglect," and plucked half of my left eyebrows out. They've still not grown back completely. "Ouch" on the vanity.)

6. Other than adjusting in rainy conditions, styling my hair has been the most difficult for me; therefore, for women with curly

hair and cowlicks, like mine, a longer, mid-length "do" works better; so the cowlicks don't own my life.

7. Also for women with only one hand, try a "new fangled volumizer." It makes styling hair much easier than a curling iron; it looks like a curling iron. Anyone can purchase it in a beauty supply shop.

8. For women and men, use a shampoo/conditioner in the shower; it saves time.

9. Find an automatic hand stamp machine in the stationery store, as well as an automatic letter opener. They have solved my envelope woes!

10. I recommend investing in a computer. There's nothing like typing letters to friends, or writing a journal to express yourself. I am doing it with one hand now, flying over the keyboard like a professional.

importance of a spouse

As was stated in the preceding stroke literature, the importance of a spouse is an important issue. As I have also expressed, my husband's help has surmounted many mountains of misery and treacherous tributaries taking me, like a hero, in his arms, over obstacles that jutted in my path along this journey. His life has changed from the sailor of yesteryear: casually cruising the oceans with no worries, no hurry, no hurricanes; only the sounds of soothing waters, slapping sails, and loving laughter; with seasoned sunshine on Sundays saved for this surrendering sensation, this pleasure. He sold his boat before my stroke, his swinger days halting. Our routine today schedules around what's easiest for him. This changed man effortlessly adapted to: selecting and orchestrating

CD morning music with the tempo suited to his mood, making the bed in the morning, drying me after my shower, aiding in my dressing, doing his bookkeeping, making necessary telephone calls, selecting a suitable restaurant to take his wife for a secluded luncheon date, marketing, combing through a collection of cookbooks, replacing bathroom readings of different material, cooking delicious dinners, inventing recipes, clearing and cleansing the glass dining table, loading and emptying the dishwasher, taking a momentary walk, creating a bedtime snack, exercising my left arm, brushing his teeth — all before midnight and late night television, all before tomorrow repeats the same routine.

My mate is a rare genuine gem. I painted this portrait to illustrate that a spouse's story has meat as well, not always following the cookbook recipe in the marriage manual of "vows", although for me the diet of love has generally become generously sprinkled with consistency. There have been ups and downs with these seasons. A marriage of substance wouldn't work if it didn't leave room for learning, growing; exercising, cultivating, practicing deeper communication skills.

Studies have varied on their statistical outcomes regarding spousal care. Some indicated that overprotectiveness can lead to dependency. Others recommended that the spouse/caregiver offer needed help, creating adjustment and progress. Other research indicated that living alone helped foster independence: that those living alone show more improvement than those who live with their spouses or other family members.[40] In essence, many studies varied in this area.

---

[40] See Thompson in the Bibliography.

importance of family

Equally important, one of the most difficult branches along this journey has been the acceptance of friends' and family members' silence. They visited me in the hospital, supported me with their smiles. This has been a receiving blessing, a gift from them to me. But sometimes in my stroke paranoia, I feel invisible. It's as though they really don't see me. No one has mentioned that I've even had a stroke, except my daughter and son — who always insists upon a two-armed hug. God bless him! I'd settle for them saying, "You've come a long way, babe; I see progress," or "What a struggle it must be for you, and Norm."

Stepson Shaun once told me he was "proud of me," when I entered graduate school. That felt very good inside. My ego needed his confirmation, his verbal approval. My stepson-in-law, playfully gruff with his comments, tries to put me down. I welcome his sadistic humor, for it indicates I'm real, here, alive for inspection, interaction, and punches. It's a delicate subject, nevertheless, one that needs emphasizing, for as was stated in the American Heart Association's literature: family and friends are one of the most important adjuncts toward healing, responsible for an adequate grieving response in the stroke patient.

Finally, it needs to be said, completing this section, that during my Attachment and Loss class, instructed by Dr. Pauline De Lozier, I received valuable and profound insights accompanied by strong feelings which in essence were: unless an earlier loss is mourned adequately, later losses accumulate, resulting in exaggerated grieving. This, supported in J. Worden's textbook, states:

Masked or repressed grief generally turns up in one of

two ways: either it is masked as a physical symptom or it is masked through some type of aberrant or maladaptive behavior. Persons who do not allow themselves to experience grief directly may develop medical symptoms similar to those which the deceased displayed or they may develop some other kind of psychosomatic complaint. For example, pain can often be a symbol for suppressed grief, or patients being treated for various somatoform disorders may have an underlying grief issue.[41]

I discuss this issue further in the Epilogue. I am reminded of my earlier comment in the History chapter that said, "These words felt like a sharp, hot knife, stabbing deep into my chest." It is also not uncanny to think of the metaphors that "someone needs strokes," which was obviously a significant issue in my life — needing "strokes" — as well as *"clawing"* my way out of this hole. I speculate, therefore, that all of my life-threatening medical problems and symptoms may be an unconscious endeavor to resolve my earlier father loss, resulting in incomplete grieving. This theory is also developed in the Epilogue.

Knowledge illuminates one's path. Bereavement cleanses the soul, washing away the debris.

---

[41] See Worden in the Bibliography.

Chapter 15

LIGHT BEYOND THE RAINBOW

Summary

AS A FINAL CHAPTER, THIS WILL ENCOMPASS A SUMMARY WITH PSYCHOLOGICAL implications, themes, generalizations, and questions for future investigators.

First, to tie in the substance of this book it is necessary to emphasize the importance of early recognition of the stroke signs highlighted in the American Heart/Stroke material. For example, the "curtain over my right eye," causing momentary darkness, was a TIA (Transient Ischemic Attack) associated with a precursor stroke. If education had been the primary focus, this may have been my life saver, preventing the forthcoming events.

Second, immediate rehabilitation is critical.

Third, the necessity of a stroke support group fulfills and

facilitates the social and psychological steps of the stroke patient following the occurrence.

Fourth, a stroke patient's spouse is a valuable link in the support chain, as are other family members and friends, each responsible for any glimmer of hope if the patient's personality radically changes from her former self, or if he or she is unable to vocalize, if aphasic. The basic issue is survival.

themes and generalizations

Depression is a common thread throughout the stroke/healing/recovery process, and can be generalized. The right and left brain hemispheres each have their own stroke characteristics generalizing their commonalties. Motivation, lack of self-esteem and confidence, are each important determinants of recovery. Additionally, patience is another vital element in the process. It takes time to heal old wounds. Scars will be evident, like favorite bookmarks, as reminders that the courage and will to heal demands patience.

Some stroke sufferers I know personally have resigned themselves to becoming slaves of silence, surrendering, giving up. I remember how long it took to eat, to dress, to feel comfortable with my new body. I pause in wonderment as I continually design this new body: visualizing, sensing the subtle changes. I'm still in this time zone that studies and marvels at how long this healing, grieving process takes — this infinitely extended journey — this intense, adventurous process of stroke survival.

I have learned, in these 10 years, to become patient with myself, and with the illusion of time. I know my unfinished business will be there for me to digest, if I wish to rehash it, amending, making friends with my childish dreams, the demons, the debris, the holes, the hurts. In other words, grieving: making peace with those who did not know better, those who were in the infancy of their becoming. To glue together these frayed ends soon becomes one's life experiences — the completed tapestry.

questions for future investigators

What then will complete the tapestry for the future investigators? What questions will impart a sense of closure, completeness? Certainly, experientially one wants to avoid a stroke, and does not need one to survey the field. Will future measurements and methods of stroke survivors' conditions be more accurate? What new treatments can a clinician offer to his or her stroke client?

Recently, I was given a treatment recovery advertisement that says: "Stroke Recovery! — 90% Improve — With Our Unique Program — The Steenblock Institute." This advertisement offers an alternative healing with the use of a hyperbaric oxygen chamber, best known for treating difficult wounds. Scuba divers with the bends and sports professionals use the chamber to decrease healing time. Interesting, but is there adequate research data offering scientific evidence this will work?

Future investigators, how would you motivate a depressed stroke client who is helplessly stranded in his intrinsic imprisonment? What quality of life can you promise a post-stroke client? What dressing strategies can you inspire for his independence? What relaxation exercises can you provide? How will you motivate encouragement? How will you inspire yourself? What subjective experience can you address that will offer hope, or courage to go beyond her shattered limits?

Included in the theme of this paper is the term *synchronicity*. The definition in The American Heritage Dictionary states: "Synchronicity—To arrange or represent so as to indicate parallel existence or occurrence." Jung gives this concept credit in his writings, having experienced this phenomenon many times himself. Also, the term *serendipity* verifies this concept, asserting: "Serendipity—the aptitude for making fortunate (accidental discoveries) is a source of important conceptual hypotheses in scientific research."[42] Therefore, within this document, as a subjective witness, I sensed an undercurrent theme of synchronicity. It may not be obvious to those whose left brain hemispheres are more linear in thinking. This consideration allows the more nonlinear thinker to reflect the meaningfulness of: "one healing phase led to another." One person dissolved, morphing into another. Moreover, I trusted the process. I touched the numinous. In my *Grief Counseling and Grief Therapy* text, by J. Worden, there is an opening quote that offers deep peace. It says: "Only people who are capable of loving strongly can also suffer great sorrow, but this same necessity of loving serves to counteract their grief and heals them."

Ultimately, throughout life, one grieves lost minutes, healing the vanishing seconds by taking with them their history. As I see in the mirror, an older, wiser, blossoming person, I rejoice in my aging process. Living is loving; loving is living. Recovery from any hazardous blow to self, loved one or addiction, is a loss — certainly stroke is a loss — and, as every loss will reflect, synthesize, and reorganize, it will eventually rest in its rightful corner. Grieving transforms healing; healing metamorphoses grieving, revolutionizing, changing forms in an endless circle. Finally, as my wise, dear

---

[42] See Matheson, et al. in the Bibliography.

father said, "Things will reveal themselves, in time." And, Daddy, wherever you are, you can pound your chest in pride, for your devoted daughter has risen from victim to victor — because of your early teachings, and love. You have shown me there is hope after stroke! I instinctively know that the light beyond the rainbow is a source that flows within my soul, and my heart.

Epilogue

RIDING THE RIM OF THE RAINBOW

analysis

THIS JOURNEY DOES NOT FEEL COMPLETE UNLESS I DISCUSS THE EXPEriences, feelings, and findings that occurred during the composing of this writing, relating with the overall theme. As there are multicolors in a rainbow, varied hues cast glows that decorate and brighten a healing process: there are many colors on a palette to select from to paint the textured portrait that completes a design.

It is imperative to help the reader understand this dissertation writing journey was not smooth. It contained many cul-de-sacs that created conflict, confusion, anxieties.

Toward the completion of writing, when I was at the point of no return, my computer program gave me problems, crashing. I thought I had lost my data, even with backup material. Norm installed a new version of my word processor. We hoped this would solve the problem. It didn't. I communicated frequently over the phone with the technical support.

This problem caused extreme anxiety. My sleep became disturbed because of it. I analyzed these feelings, evaluating the implications.

The major fear stemmed from loss; loss beyond the printed page. Symbolically, this document represents my being — my whole, reconstructed, healed self — the reason I was born. Thus, losing it was the worst, negative nightmare; a scenario I wanted to escape. This meant I would have lost my "self": the whole, independent "self" I had striven unconsciously, consciously, and conscientiously to create.

The bottom level suggests survival versus demise. The mere thought of this potential mega-loss triggers trembling from an inner part of my being.

The psychological therapeutic power from this paper has been the realization that I never thoroughly grieved for my original, deep loss: my father's death. I became aware of this when reading the final chapter of this paper. At the conclusion, I found myself sobbing, uncontrollably, without restraint. It occurred to me that I had not grieved. It appeared not allowed. It seemed prohibited, not encouraged. As an 8-year-old child, I saw no tears from my mother. There were no loving arms to hold me; no spoken words that comforted or inquired about feelings or thoughts. This need was real, albeit absent. I do not intend for this to amplify as a "poor little me" saga; for others have weathered far stronger storms and survived.

Consequently, each subsequent loss in my life piled up, reading like lines from Carl Sandburg's poem that says, "Pile box on box and the bottom box says; 'it all rests on me.'"

attachment and loss theory

John Bowlby, the master therapist who developed his Attachment and Loss Theory, suggests a reasonable thesis regarding my situation. He states: "For, as children know in their bones, when mother is prone to be rejecting it may be better to placate her than to risk alienating her altogether."[43]

This states my position, exactly.

Moreover, Bowlby indicates there are certain classes of events that can act as "precipitants of breakdown" during a loss. One of his four categories includes reaching the same age as was a parent when he or she died. My father died at 49; I was 48 when my life-threatening crisis occurred. Although I did not consciously know his age of demise until a few years ago, I ponder Bowlby's position along this line. Was it coincidence, or another synchronicity? "Another archetype of magical effect, a universal trait in all humans," as Carl Jung recognized.

Bowlby also alludes to the fact that "threats of abandonment create as much anxiety as actual abandonment." This becomes apparent from studying my flashbacks: the disappearance of the green Chevrolet as a young child; the "San Francisco episode"; the tearful reaction in the shoe department, when Norm whispered his "dumb" aside.

It is also my theory that my physical illnesses appeared unconsciously created, or caused, as an inner anger, which I thrust upon myself and symbolically structured "deep within." Although speculative, evidence supports this, as one of the many abnormal grief reactions is masked grief reaction. "Masked grief reactions are

---

[43] See Bowlby in the Bibliography.

interesting in that patients experience symptoms and behaviors that cause them difficulty but do not see or recognize the fact that these relate to the loss."[44]

Bowlby's thesis is that early attachments come from a need for security and safety; they develop early in life, and are usually directed toward a few specific individuals, and tend to endure throughout a large part of the life cycle.

When my father's death occurred, I entered the three stages Bowlby postulates: "protest, despair, detachment." However, these were on an unconscious level, using Bowlby's term, "defensive exclusion."

Bowlby also states, "the biological disequilibrium brought about by the sudden change in the environment which influences grieving; can be compared in the same way they have been for wounds, burns, and infections"

grief therapy

Bowlby sequences four key phases of mourning. They are:

1. Phase of numbing that usually lasts from a few hours to a week and may be interrupted by outbursts of extremely intense distress and/or anger.

2. Phase of yearning and searching for the lost figure lasting some months and sometimes for years.

3. Phase of disorganization and despair.

4. Phase of greater or lesser degree of reorganization.

In addition, knowing this information as an adult, it is noteworthy to establish today's healthy reality by understanding the

---

[44] See Worden in the Bibliography.

Four Tasks of Mourning. These are the tasks one must go through to achieve complete mourning.

Task I: To accept the reality of the loss.

Task II: To work through to the pain of grief.

Task III: To adjust to an environment in which the deceased is missing.

Task IV: To emotionally relocate the deceased and move on with life.[45]

It is also helpful to become aware of six myths we, as a society, teach regarding grieving. They are:

1. Bury your feelings.
2. Replace the loss.
3. Grieve alone.
4. Just give it time.
5. Regret the past (*Different, Better, or More*).
6. Don't trust.[46]

As an adult, as a student, I apply this wisdom in my current life; and will teach this to others in need, as part of my "mission."

conclusion

Cerebrovascular accident, or stroke, is a serious health problem, striking as many as 600,000 people in the United States each year. Those who survive the initial incident are often left with a

---

[45] See Worden in the Bibliography.
[46] See James and Cherry in the Bibliography.

variety of medical problems, including hemiplegia, cognitive deficits, and speech dysfunction. This book strives to educate and enlighten the reader in a nonstatistical, qualitative format, taking advantage of my personal stroke in this 10-year narrative, detailing the process of post-stroke recovery, augmented with scientific evidence substantiating my journey. In this approach, I attempted to address treatments consisting of physical, speech and occupational rehabilitation programs designed to help the patient recover lost functioning.

In addition to physical disability, stroke patients are likely to experience a variety of psychological problems arising from concerns about their present plight. These include feelings of loss of control, fears about death and disfigurement, social isolation, helplessness, and worry about the loss of social roles and everyday existence.

Depression and emotional instability are common reactions. These concerns are felt by the families who are faced with the prospect of long-term care, financial and emotional strain, as well as quality of life in the years following the stroke. Adjustment, adaptation, coping, rehabilitation, feeling stigmatized or supported and wanted are major issues plaguing the stroke survivor. Finding meaningfulness in the domain of this shattered life becomes a treasured word. But the most cherished word the stroke survivor clings to is, H O P E.

I end with two meaningful quotations:

"The quiet 'little deaths' of everyday existence are mourned as much as those of resounding magnitude, for grief makes no comparisons nor judgments, and has no understanding of degree."[47]

---

[47] See Berkus in the Bibliography.

And last, "a thing which has not been understood inevitably reappears; like an unlaid ghost, it cannot rest until the mystery has been resolved and the spell broken" (Sigmund Freud).

On March 21, 1995, my 10-year-stroke anniversary, the mystery resolved and the spell broke. I am currently riding the rim of the rainbow, as my journey continues on the wings of hope. For "Hope gives us wings to rise above life's disappointments to the blue sky that is always waiting just beyond the clouds." Indeed, there is hope after stroke! Thus, the triumph of human spirit.

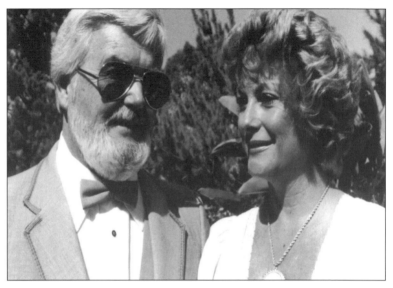

Marty and Norm, before Emmy Ceremony in the early 1970s.

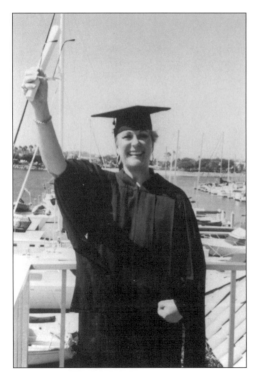

Marty receiving Master of Arts Degree in 1994.

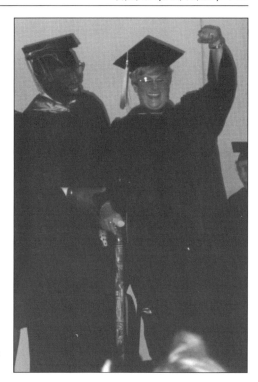

Marty receiving Doctorate; Claw celebrates too.

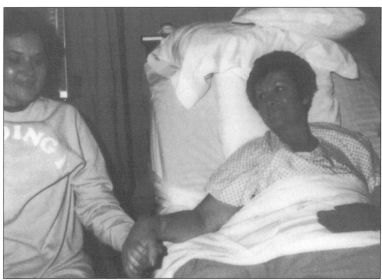

Marty, in hospital following stroke, with roomate Susan.

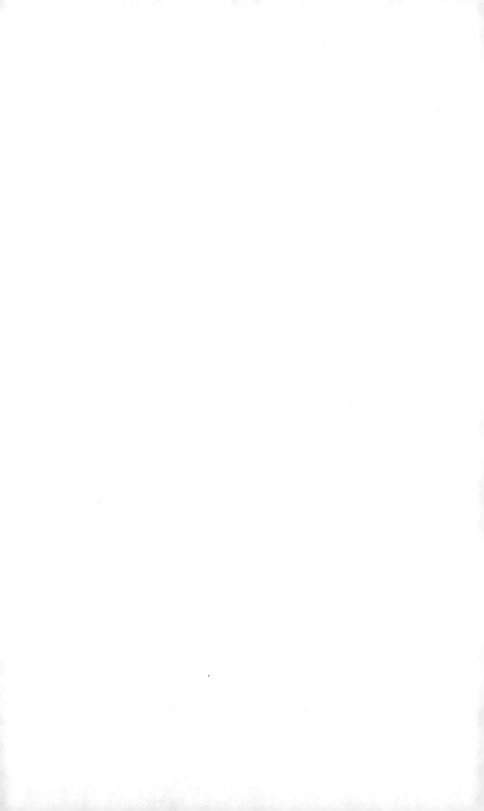

A Final Essay: The Cane, Graduation, the Doctor and the Gift

As an afterthought, to feel complete in my stroke journey, I wish to share with the readers the finale in achieving my doctorate — the greatest achievement in my life thus far. It begins with a phone call.

It was Saturday. Norm and I listened to a soft-spoken female phone message saying, "Hi, I'm Nicky from the Florist and I have an order for you and can't find your street in the Thomas guide. My number is 822-5900. Please call and I'll deliver it." I replayed the sweet-sounding voice three times; each time it said the same thing. Norm was beginning to enjoy the sensual female tones, wondering if she had a 900 number! I called the number. A computer voice told me that number was no longer in service, "please check your number or try again." I tried again. Same message. I hung up wondering who was Nicky with the sweet-sounding voice, who was the florist, and who was the order from. It was a mystery I longed to resolve; but let it go; and laid my swollen, broken, now in a cast, foot down on the higher-than-my-heart two pillows. I gulped prescribed pain pills one after another followed by Tylenol; meditated, then prepared for the BIG DR day — my doctoral graduation.

I was elevating my [paralyzed] swollen left foot, having broken it on a Thursday, ten days prior to this major lifetime graduation. It was a nightmare I wish I could forget. But it still haunts my memory.

I had tripped on my daughter's giant overnight duffel bag, when she was visiting. I was in shock, while witnessing my body in slow motion as I fell to the floor, landing on her stuffed bag, my foot awkwardly bent, like a broken crayon, stuck underneath my bottom. Earlier, I had told myself while maneuvering around the pull-out sofa-bed, "I must be very careful and not trip on her bag." As soon as I said this, down I went, unable to stand up by myself. Moaning, I screeched for Norm to help me up, as it was impossible to get up myself, even though this had been one hospital/rehab lesson. He and my daughter came running to my aid immediately.

Ignoring the instantaneous swelling the foot displayed, Norm and I left our home to lead the Stroke Support Group in our area. I hobbled as I tried to walk from the car to the building. I asked Norm to get a wheelchair at the entrance of the senior center. By now, it was impossible to walk on my swollen, painful foot. The wheelchair was a luxury, and I remembered my former hospital wheelchair experiences.

Eventually, we went to the emergency hospital after the

conclusion of the stroke group, after dinner. My foot was X-rayed, pronounced broken, and put into a cast. "A six-week recovery period" was told to me by one in the emergency team. My doctoral graduation in a cast? I groaned. Norm said something like, "And there goes my weekends!" Visualizing having to help me — even more. I think I laughed at his bittersweet response.

I now needed a cane. I had recycled my earlier hospital stroke cane, giving it to my father-in-law, Oliver. The only cane I had was my mother's. It was flimsy. I told Norm I'd like a new, sturdier cane to help my balance. My late mother's cane, which I used for a day, was about as strong as a tree branch that had fallen in the wind. We scouted the drug stores and medical supplies but all their fancy canes were $80+! Forget that; I'd use Mother's tree branch.

When Consuelo, our housecleaning artist, saw my flimsy cane, she said she had a very sturdy one her brother found while working in an airport. Someone from El Salvador left it, and it was now in her storage/garage. Bless her kind, gentle heart; she delivered it to me on Saturday, and what a cane! It is a decorator's dream: hand carved in primitive Egyptian/Mayan/South American-like art, the face and head bare snarling, sharp teeth, and pointed black and red ears. It's probably worth a fortune. At least to me it is. Thick and sturdy, and a designer's dream to boot. "What Marta wants, Marta gets!" I've christened him "Beauty," or perhaps "Beast," depending upon my mood. There were six people in the mall who commented on it as I strolled through following our haircutting appointment. While holding it in my right hand, walking on the mall's marble floor, I felt secure, balanced.

Yet I still fretted about graduation and walking in the procession and onto the stage.

The big DR graduation day came calmly. It was a success. We

arrived early. Because of my broken foot, and knowing I was unable to walk up the outside steps with my graduate colleagues, I waited in the back of the Marina room, watching from the windows San Diego Sunday sailboats drifting in the distance thinking I was in San Francisco. I sat quietly, perched like a lost, wounded bird by the side, breezy, entrance door where all the graduates would soon enter. I reflected as I waited, observing, as Roseanne and Patty puttered around doing their last minute party organizing. The starting time approached quicker than Cinderella's midnight carriage.

My friend Jean put my flat yellow-tasseled graduation hat on my head, fastening it with bobbypins, flattening my sassy new hairstyle like a pancake. I prayed it would pouf up properly, later. (It did.) Jean also helped me put on my black graduation gown over my black skirt and black Velcro cast. Immediately, the gown's zipper broke. Panic. We were in a hurry. The other graduates were assembling, ready to march up the huge, steep iron stairs outside the breezy door. Norm said he could fix the faulty zipper. Fumbling with his hurry-up hands, he finally mastered clamping the zipper's bottom, silver pull, doodad that had fallen off onto the floor. Using his teeth he said, "I'll use my pliers later at home." Relief. Familiar faces graced my landscape, greeting me, smiling, soon finding a seat to view this grand parade.

The graduates appeared in the doorway. The swift breeze seemed to settle. The music started with a jerk, sounding as if the record needle was stuck. Suddenly I remembered I was told to put my doctoral hood over my left stroke arm. I tried to obey this request. It kept sliding off the smooth, slippery, sleeve surface. Quickly, my sister solved the problem. She stuck it under my stubborn, stiff stroke thumb; and I was soon joining the procession, connecting the thread ahead of classmate, Cherlynn; grasping my breath; and the decorated cane in my right hand, doctoral hood now fixed under the left thumb.

My thoughts raced. Will I make it to my seat? Will my broken foot/cast trip on one of the aisle chairs? Will my hood fall from my stuck thumb? Instant fear. "Relax," my inner voice spoke. "Go with the flow."

At my seat I smiled broadly, feeling pride, as I saw family and dear friends sitting like proper little soldiers in the front rows, each with their black cameras focused on my thoughts, on my proud face puffed up from pain pills. I waved inside, listening to speeches of being a Good Samaritan in the community. I thought of brother-in-law, Tony; he is always the Good Samaritan. I listened to my classmate describe what I'm going through with internship woes, the economy, using creativity, hope, for the future challenge. Yes, hope I thought. There is hope!

The speeches and ceremony faded like a dream. It ended softly like a curtain closing across my mind. When it was my turn to become degreed, I felt strong support under both arms, while aided up the originally feared rickety stairs, onto the stage, by the two gallant professors. I saw my doctoral hood, wrinkled now from squeezing it so tightly, being taken from my tightly clasped thumb and felt its taffeta and velvet purple glow slide — over the head it went — I was Dr. M. Otto Hopps! I had climbed the mountain!

Facing the multitude, I saluted this thrill by raising Claw — my stroke arm — with the rhythm of a boxing champion, which I had been practicing for eleven years! Up it came, albeit shaky. I heard myself yell, "Hooray!" I heard cheers. I saw tears sparkling in the shadows.

I thought to myself, one broken foot, two giant leaps into a new beginning with a strong belief: with creativity, and with hope, I've made it this far, I'll surely make it all the way — to the state licensing mountaintop — as another Good Samaritan along the way.

The aftermath on Monday was really the celebration. As I put my treasured gifts away I answered the telephone call. It was Nicky, the florist with the sweet, sensual voice from the anonymous shop. "Will you be home in an hour?" Yes, I answered.

I opened the door to a very pretty young woman in cutoff blue jeans reaching out with the most delicate bouquet in a basket that had rainbow-colored flowers resembling the "Angel Pat" aura. It was definitely a Koethian arrangement: a loving gift by two very special friends. Norm was in the shower so he wasn't able to see who Nicky with the soft-spoken voice belonged to. Too bad. Maybe that's why he's hinting about a 900 number. Perhaps next year.

And, I continue my journey farther, even though I've fallen while on a neighborhood walk a couple of times. Although resulting in bruised knees like a child, I practice picking myself up, *knowing* there are tests that teach me: with practice, perseverance, and most of all patience, I will continue the triumph of human spirit. It is all in the hands of hope. My hand. This is the true gift. Yes, the gift of hope, and the satisfaction of believing, *knowing* — and trusting the process.

Glossary of Stroke-Related Medical Terms

Achilles tendon: The powerful tendon at the back of the heel formed by the united tendons of the large muscles of the calf.

Adrenal cortex: Part of adrenal gland that secretes hormones affecting growth and gonads.

Agnosia: Loss of the ability to recognize sensory impressions, especially of touch, sight, and hearing.

Aneurysm: Dilation of a segment of a blood vessel, often involving the aorta or pulmonary artery.

Angiogram: An X-ray photograph of blood vessels after an injection of a radiopaque substance.

Aorta: Great artery arising from left ventricle, carrying blood from the heart to all parts of the body.

Aphasia: The loss or reduction of the ability to speak, read, write, or understand, due to dysfunction of brain centers.

Apoplexy: Stroke.

Aspiration pneumonia: Pneumonia caused by inhaling foreign matter into the lungs. Most aspiration pneumonia in stroke survivors is caused by inhaling food or drink into the lungs, usually as the result of impaired swallowing ability.

Blood-thinning medication: Drugs designed to prevent the formation or further growth of blood clots. These drugs work by interfering with one or more of the blood components or processes essential to the clotting process.

Brain stem: The stemlike part of the brain that connects the brain's right and left hemispheres with the spinal cord. Responsible for nonthinking activities such as breathing, blood pressure, and coordination of eye movements.

Carotid artery: An artery that carries blood from the heart to the brain. One can have a carotid artery on each side of your neck. Each artery divides into "internal" and "external" carotid arteries. Each external carotid artery supplies blood to the neck and face. Each internal carotid supplies blood to the front part of the brain.

Carotid endarterectomy: The surgical removal of the lining of a carotid artery. Performed when the artery is significantly diseased or blocked.

Cerebellum: The second largest portion of the brain, responsible for coordinating voluntary muscle movements.

Cerebral edema: Swelling of the brain due to an increase in its water content.

Contracture: A permanent shortening of muscle, tendon, or ligament.

CT or "CAT" scanner: A specialized form of X-ray that allows physicians to see the internal structure of the brain in precise detail.

CVA: Cerebrovascular Attack: Stroke.

Dysphagia: Inability to or difficulty in swallowing.

Electrocardiogram (ECG or EKG): A recording of the electrical activity of the heart.

Electroencephalogram: The record produced by tracing of

brain waves by means of electrodes on the scalp or in the brain itself.

Embolic stroke: A stroke resulting from the blockage of an artery by a blood clot (or "embolus").

Embolism: Term used to describe the blockage of a blood vessel by a blood clot.

Embolus: A mass of undissolved matter in a blood vessel, carried there by the bloodstream. In the case of stroke, the undissolved matter is usually a blood clot.

Emotionally lability: Instability or changeability of the emotions. In stroke survivors, emotional lability usually takes the form of inappropriate laughing or crying (i.e., for no obvious reason).

Foot drop: Inability to pull the foot and toes up toward the shin. Common in patients who are in bed continuously (especially if comatose). Can usually be prevented through the use of a footboard.

Heart attack: Death of heart tissue caused by the blockage of one or more of the arteries supplying blood to the heart. Also called a myocardial infarction.

Hemiparesis: Paralysis affecting only one side of the body.

Hemorrhagic stroke: A stroke caused by a ruptured blood vessel and characterized by bleeding within or surrounding the brain.

Hypesthesia: A diminished tactile sensibility that interferes with the ability to feel the results of a runny nose on the hemiplegic side.

Impairment: A difficulty in performing or lack of ability to perform an action. In stroke, an impairment is generally the direct result of damage to an area of the brain controlling a specific action. Sometimes referred to as a "neurological deficit."

Infarct (Infarction): Brain injury, or damage.

Intravenous: Within a vein.

Left hemisphere: The left half of the brain. Controls the actions of the right side of the body, as well as analytic abilities, such as calculating, speaking and writing.

Left-side neglect: A lack of awareness of actions or objects on the left side of the body. For example, a stroke survivor with left-side neglect may ignore or forget about food on the left side of the dinner plate. To help this person, remind him or her about the left side of the plate, or move the food to the right side of the plate.

Neurological deficit: See Impairment.

Occlusion: Obstruction of the flow of blood.

Occupational therapy: Therapy designed to help stroke survivors become independent in their activities of daily living, such as eating, bathing, and using the bathroom.

Physical therapy: Therapy which uses physical agents such as heat, massage, hydrotherapy, radiation, electricity and exercise to help patients improve or regain muscle function or strength.

Pulmonary embolism: The blockage of a lung artery by a mass of undissolved matter (usually a blood clot).

Recurrent stroke: A second or any subsequent stroke following a first stroke.

Right hemisphere: The right half of the brain. Controls the actions of the left side of the body.

Second stroke: See Recurrent stroke.

Speech and language therapy: Therapy designed to diagnose and treat defects and disorders of the voice and of spoken and written communication.

Thrombosis: The blockage of a blood vessel which is caused by the gradual buildup of deposits, with the blockage made complete when a blood clot develops on top of previously built-up deposits.

Urinary tract complications: Term used to describe a broad range of problems associated with the elimination of urine from the body. In stroke, most urinary tract complications are the result of brain and the bladder. As a result, stroke survivors may often be unable to control the elimination of urine or may retain too much urine. Physicians and nurses have a variety of ways to help stroke survivors cope with and gain control over urinary tract complications.

Vertebrobasilar artery: Artery which supplies blood to the brain stem and cerebellum.

Bibliography

American Heart Association (1995). Strokes: *A Guide for the Family.* Dallas, TX.

Beckson, M. and Cummings, J.L., Neuropsychiatric Aspects of Stroke, *Int'L. Journal Psychiatry in Medicine,* Vol. 21 (1) pp. 1-15, 1991 ("Pharmacotherapy has proved useful in post stroke depression" and ". . . patients with the abrupt onset of delusions and auditory, visual and tactile hallucinations following right temporoparietal infarctions").

Bell, E., Jurek, K. & Wilson, T.: Hand skill measurement. *Am J Occup Ther* 30: 80-86, 1976.

Berkus, R. (1984). *To Heal Again.* California: Red Rose Press.

Berthier, M., and. Starkstein S.E., Acute atypical psychosis following a right hemisphere stroke, *Acta Neurogica Belgica,* 87, pp. 125-131, 1987.

Birket-Smith, M., Knudsen, H.C., Nissen, J., Blegvad, N., Kohler, O., Rasmussen, D., Petersem, S. W., Life events and social support in prediction of stroke outcome. *Psychother Psychosom,* 52: pp, 146-150, 1989.

Bjorneby, E.R., and Reinvang, I.R., Acquiring and maintaining self-care skills after stroke: the predictive value of apraxia. *Scan J Rehab Med* 17: 75-80, 1985.

Bolen, J.S. (1979). *The Tao of Psychology: Synchronicity and the Self*. San Francisco: Harper/Collins.

Bowlby, J. (1980).*Vol. III: Loss Sadness and Depression*. New York: Harper/Collins.

Bowlby, J. (1988). *A Secure Base*. New York: Harper/Collins.

Breggin, P.R. (1994). *Talking Back to Prozac*. New York: St. Martin's Press.

Brocklehurst, J.P., Morris, K. Andrews, B., Richards, and P. Laycock, 'Social effects of stroke.' *Social Science and Medicine*, 15a: 35-9., 1981.

Calvanio, R., Levine, D., Petrone, P., Elements of cognitive rehabilitation after right hemisphere stroke. *Behavioral Neurology*, Vol. 11 n1, pp. 25-53, 1993.

Champeau, T., Transactional Analysis in stroke rehabilitation: TA and medical practice. *Transactional Analysis Journal*. Vol. 13, No. 1, pp. 50-54, 1983.

Croisile B., Tourniare C., Confavreux, et al., Bilateral damage to the head of the caudate nuclei, *Annals of Neurology*. 25, pp. 313-314, 1989.

Diller, L., Buxbaum, J. & Chiotelis, S.: Relearning motor skills in hemiplegia: Error analysis. *Genet Psychol Monogr* 85: 249-286, 1972.

Eastwood M. R., Rifat, Hobbs S., et al., Mood disorder following Cerebrovascular accident, *British Journal of Psychiatry*, 154, pp. 195-200, 1989.

Ebrahim, S., Barer, D., Nouri, F., Affective Illness after stroke. *British Journal of Psychiatry*, 151, pp. 52-56, 1987.

Evans, R.L., and Miller, R.M., Psychosocial implications and treatment of stroke: In News and Views, *Social Casework: The Journal of Contemporary Social Work*, 65 (n4) pp. 242-247,1984.

Feinberg, T.E. and Shapiro, R.M., Misidentification-Reduplication and the right hemisphere, *Neuropsychology, and Behavioral Neurology*, 2, pp. 39-48, 1989.

Finklestein, S., Benowitz, L. I., Baldessarini, R., et al., Mood, vegetative disturbance, and dexamethasone suppression test after stroke, *Annals of Neurology*, 12, pp. 463-468, 1982.

Garrity, T.F. Vocational adjustment after first myocardial infarction; Comparative assessment of several variables suggested in the literature. *Social Science and Medicine*, 7, pp. 705-717,1973.

Gray, J. (1992). *Men are from Mars, Women are from Venus.* New York: Harper/Collins.

Hachinski, V: Stroke rehabilitation. *Archives of Neurology* 46: p.703, 1989 ("Few areas in neurology are in greater need of critical examination than stroke rehabilitation. . . . Isaac's lament has not been redressed, 'Experts in stroke rehabilitation abound, but none of them has proven anything about rehabilitation to the satisfaction of anyone else'" (p. 703).

Henley, S., Pettit, S., Todd-Pokropek, A., Tupper, A.M., Who goes home? Predictive factors in stroke recovery. *Journal of Neurology, and Psychiatry*, 48: pp. 1-6, 1985 ("In most cases the therapists, who also had discussions with the nursing staff, had no difficulty in deciding whether or not a patient was well motivated towards his rehabilitation" (p. 2)).

Hier, D.B., Mondlock, B.A., & Callan, L.R., Recovery of behavioral abnormalities after right hemisphere stroke. *Neurology;* 33: pp. 345-50, 1983.

Holroyd. Pushing the limits of recovery: Hypnotherapy with a stroke patient. *International Journal of Clinical Hypnosis*, Apr., v 37,n2, pp. 120-128, (1989).

Hyman, M.D. Disability and patients' perceptions of preferential treatment: Some preliminary findings. *Journal of Chronic Diseases*. 24, pp. 329-342,1971.

James, J. & Cherry, F. (1988). *The Grief Recovery Handbook*. New York: Harper/Collins.

Joy, B. (1979). *Joy's Way*. Los Angeles: J.P. Tarcher.

Jung, C.G. (1989). *Memories, Dreams, Reflections*. (Ed)., Jaffe, A. New York: Random House.

Klawans, H.L. (1990). *Newton's Madness: Further Tales of Clinical Neurology*. New York: Harper/Row.

Kolb, B. Recovery from occipital stroke: A self-report and an inquiry into visual processes. *Canadian Journal of Psychology*, 44(2), pp. 130-147, 1990.

Kramer, P.D.(1993). *Listening to Prozac*. New York: Penguin Books.

Kubler-Ross, E.(1986). *Death: The Final Stage of Growth*. New York: Simon & Schuster.

Lincoln, N.B., Blackburn, M., Ellis, S., Jackson, J.J., Edmans, J.A., Nouri, F.M., Walrer, M.F., Haworth, H., An investigation of factors affecting progress of patients on a stroke unit. *Journal of Neurology, and Psychiatry*; 52: pp. 493-496, 1989.

Lipsey R., Robinson, R.G., Pearlson, et al., Nortripyline treatment of post-stroke depression: A double-blind study, *The Lancet*, 84, pp. 297-300, 1984.

Matheson, Bruce, Beauchamp, 1978. *Experimental Psychology: Research Designs and Analysis*.(3rd ed). Florida: Holt, Rinehart, & Winston.

Meerwaldt, J.D., Spatial disorientation in right-hemisphere infarction: a study of the speed of recovery. *Journal of Neurology, Neurosurgery, and Psychiatry*, 46: pp. 426-129, 1983 ("Recovery mainly took place in the first six months after the stroke. Most patients then performed at a normal level. A relation between the size of the lesion (assessed from CT scans) and the speed of recovery was found." (p. 426)).

Messner, M., and Messner, E., Mood disorder following stroke. *Comprehensive Psychiatry*, Vol. 29, n1(Jan/Feb., pp. 22-27, 1988 ("Aprosodic voice patterns may simulate flattened affect, and the clinician may disbelieve his reports of dysphoria. On the other hand, a flattened affect does not necessarily indicate depression" (p. 23) and "A Cerebrovascular accident has many disturbing effects such as worry about recurrence, loss of control, insanity, and even death—all of which easily lends itself to a psychological explanation of depression" (p. 22)).

Morris, P.,L.P., Robinson, R.G., Raphael, B., Bishop, D., The relationship between the perception of social support and post-stroke depression in hospitalized patients. *Psychiatry*, Vol. 54, pp. 306-315,1991 ("If patients perceive inadequate support from their spouse, the ensuing insult to self-esteem and sense of abandonment may have particular salience, resulting in depressive symptoms (p. 313).").

National Stroke Association,(1995). Stroke (Prevention): The Brain at risk—Understanding and preventing stroke. Colorado: *National Stroke Association*.

National Stroke Association,(1995). Stroke: (Survivor & Caretaker Resources): Living at home after a stroke. Colorado: *National Stroke Association*.

National Stroke Association,(1995). Stroke (Acute care): Stroke treatment & recovery. Colorado: *National Stroke Association*.

Newman, S. The social and emotional consequences of head injury and stroke. *International Review of Applied Psychology*, Vol. 33

pp. 427-55, 1984 ("Goldstein's view was that the Catastrophic Reaction was particularly evident when the patient was taxed beyond his abilities" (p. 443) and "With regard to neurotic conditions, anxiety states including phobia, hypochondriasis, obsessive neurosis, general irritability and various somatic complaints have been found to follow head injury" (p. 436).

Norris, V.K., Stephens, MA Parris, Kinney, J.M., Impact of Family interactions on recovery from stroke: Help or hindrance? *Gerontologist*, Vol. 30; (n4): pp. 535-542, 1990.

Panzeri, M., Semenza, C., & Butterworth, B., Compensatory processes in the evolution of severe jargon aphasia. *Neuropsychologia*, Vol. 25, No. 6, pp. 919-933, 1987.

Perani, D., Vallar, G., Paulesu, E., Alberoni, M., & Fazio, F., Left and right hemisphere contribution to recovery from neglect after right hemisphere damage—a PET (positron emission tomography) study of two cases. *Neuropsychologia*, Vol. 31, No. 2, pp. 115-125, 1993.

Peroutka, B., Sohmer, A.J., Kumar, et al., Hallucinations and delusions following a right temporoparietooccipital infarction, *The Johns Hopkins Medical Journal*, 151, pp. 181-185, 1982.

Pickersgill, M.J., Lincoln, N.B., Prognostic indicators and the pattern of recovery of communication in aphasic stroke patients. *Journal of Neurology, Neurosurgery, and Psychiatry*, 46: pp. 130-139, 1983.

Pinel, J. (1993). *Biopsychology* (2nd ed). Boston: Simon & Schuster.

Redfield, J. and Adrienne, C. (1995). *The Celestine Prophecy: An Experiential Guide*. New York: Time/Warner.

Reding M.J., Orto, L.A., Winter, S. W., et al., Antidepressant therapy after Stroke: A double-blind trial, *Archives of Neurology*, 43, pp. 763-765, 1986. "In another prospective double-blind study, trazodone was found to be associated with a greater trend toward improvement than placebo."

Robinson, R.G., Starr, L.B.,. Kubos, K.L, et al., A two year longitudinal study of post-stroke mood disorder: Findings during the initial evaluation, *Stroke*, 14, pp. 736-741, 1983 ("Previous investigations have demonstrated that post-stroke depression can adversely affect resumption of social activities, but the effect of diagnosed depression on long-term recovery from physical impairment has never been examined" (p. 785)).

Robinson, R.G., Lipsey, J.R., Fedoroff, P., Price, T.R., Impact of post-stroke depression on recovery in activities of daily living over a 2-year follow-up. *Arch Neurology*, Vol. 47, pp. 785-789, 1990.

Ross, E.D.: The aprosodias: functional-anatomic organization of the effective components of language in the right hemisphere. *Archives of Neurology* 38:561-569,1981 ("alterations of behavior and affective language called 'aprosodia,' which often results from lesions of the right hemisphere may confuse the clinical presentation." (p. 22)).

Ross, E.D., Rush, A.J.: Diagnosis and neuroanatomical correlates of depression in brain damaged patients. *Arch Gen Psychiatry* 38: 1344-1354, 1981.

Sacks,O. (1985). *The Man Who Mistook his Wife for a Hat and Other Clinical Tales*. New York: Summit Books.

Sarno, M.T., & Levita, E., Some observations on the nature of recovery in Global aphasia after stroke. *Brain and Language*. 13, pp. 1-12,1981.

Schiller, L., Bennett, A.,(1994). *The Quiet Room: A Journey Out of the Torment of Madness*. New York: Warner Books.

Sheehy, G. (1992). *The Silent Passage: Menopause*. New York: Random House.

Shemel'kov, V.N., Restoration of motor function in stroke patients: Peculiarities relating to damage of the right or left hemisphere. *Neurology & Behavioral Physiology*, Vol. 12 (n2): pp. 96-100, 1982 ("Differences in the way a patient regards his defect and its correction may affect the course of his rehabilitation, when the foci are located in different hemispheres of the brain." (p. 96)).

Stephens, M.A., Norris, V., and Kinney, J.M., Ritchie, S.W., Social networks and liabilities in recovery from stroke by geriatric patients. *Psychology and Aging* Vol. 2, No. 2, pp. 125-129, 1987.

The Family Therapy Networker. Psychotherapy's third wave? — The promise of narrative. (1994: November/December).

Thompson, S.C., Sobolew-Shubin, A., Graham, M.A., & Janigian, A., Psychosocial adjustment following a stroke. *Soc. Sci. Med.* Vol. 28, No. 3, pp. 239-247, 1989 (" Maintaining self-esteem is a crucial factor in speed of recovery as well as motivation" (p. 240) and "...A number of patients mentioned that having the stroke had caused them to reevaluate their priorities and to appreciate areas of their life that they had formally taken for granted. The impression that one gets from these comments is not that merely because these patients were not depressed, they saw meaning in the experience, but that some active learning or reevaluation had taken place so that they saw their life differently than they had prior to the stroke. It may be the case that this change in perspective is easier to obtain if one is not depressed" (page 245)).

Vallar, G., Perani, D., Cappa, S.F., Messa, C., Lenzi, G.L., Frazio, F., Recovery from aphasia and neglect after subcortical stroke: neuropsychological and cerebral perfusion study. *Journal of Neurology, Neurosurgery, and Psychiatry*, 51: pp. 1269-1276, 1988.

Veith, I. (1988). *Can You Hear the Clapping of One Hand?:*

Learning to Live With a Stroke. Berkeley: University of California Press.

Wade, D.T., Wood, V.A., Hewer, R.L., Recovery after stroke—The first 3 months. *Journal of Neurology, and Psychiatry*, 48: pp. 7-13, 1985.

Walker, M.F., Lincoln, N.B., Factors influencing dressing performance after stroke. *Journal of Neurology, Neurosurgery & Psychiatry*, Aug., v54 (n8):pp. 699-701,1991.

Warren, M., Relationship of constructional apraxia and body scheme disorders to dressing performance in adult CVA. *Am J Occ Therapy* 35 : (7):pp. 431-7,1981.

Williams, N.: Correlations between coping ability and dressing activities in hemiplegia. *Am J Phys Med* 46: 1332-1340, 1967.

Worden, J. (1991). *Grief Counseling & Grief Therapy: A Handbook for the Mental Health Practitioner*. New York: Springer Publishing Co.

Wortman, C. B.,& Lehman, D.R. Reactions to victims of life crises: Support attempts that fail. In I.G. Sarason & Sarason (Eds.), *Social Support: Theory, Research and Applications* (pp. 463-490),1985. The Hague, The Netherlands: Martinus Nijhoff.

Yudofsky, S., Hales, R. Ferguson, T.(1991). *What You Need to Know About Psychiatric Drugs*. New York: Ballantine Books.

Appendix

National Stroke Association
96 Inverness Drive East, Suite 1
Englewood, Colorado 80112
Web Site: www.stroke.org

Ischemic Stroke

In everyday life, blood clotting is beneficial. When one bleeds from a wound, blood clots work to slow and eventually stop the bleeding. In the case of stroke, however, blood clots are dangerous because they can block arteries and cut off blood flow.

There are two ways that a blood-clot stroke can occur.

• Embolic Stroke - The first type of blood clot stroke is when a blood clot forms somewhere in the body (usually the heart) and travels through the bloodstream to the brain. Once in the brain, the clot eventually travels to a blood vessel that's too small for it to pass through. It lodges there, blocking the blood vessel and causing a stroke. These kinds of strokes are called *embolic* strokes. The medical word for this type of blood clot is *embolus*. Blood-clot strokes can also happen as the result of unhealthy blood vessels clogged with a buildup of fatty deposits and cholesterol. The body regards these buildups as multiple, tiny, and repeated injuries to the blood vessel wall. So the body reacts to these injuries just as it would if you were bleeding from a wound — it responds by forming clots.

• Thrombotic Stroke - In the second type of blood-clot stroke, clots form around pieces of blood vessel deposits. These clots can grow big enough to block the blood vessel completely. Strokes caused in this way are called *thrombotic* strokes. That's because the medical word for a clot that forms on a blood vessel deposit is *thrombus*.

Hemorrhagic Stroke

Strokes caused by the breakage or "blowout" of a blood vessel are called hemorrhagic strokes. The medical word for this type of breakage is *hemorrhage*. Hemorrhages can be caused by a number of disorders which affect the blood vessels, including long-standing high blood pressure and cerebral aneurysms.

An *aneurysm* is a weak or thin spot on a blood vessel wall. The weak spots that cause aneurysms are usually present at birth. Aneurysms develop over a number of years and usually don't cause detectable problems until they break (National Stroke Association, 1994).

Right Hemisphere Stroke

The right hemisphere of the brain controls the movement of the left side of the body. It also controls analytical and perceptual tasks, such as judging distance, size, speed, or position, and seeing how parts are connected to wholes.

A stroke in the right hemisphere often causes paralysis in the left side of the body. This is known as *left hemiplegia*.

People who have had a right-hemisphere stroke may also have problems with their spatial and perceptual abilities. This may cause them to misjudge distances (leading to a fall) or be unable to guide their hands to pick up an object, button a shirt, or tie their shoes. They may get lost easily. Our society puts so much emphasis on communication abilities (controlled by the left hemisphere), that spatial and perceptual impairments can easily be overlooked.

Along with impaired ability to judge spatial relationships, people who have had a right-hemisphere stroke often have judgment difficulties that show up in their behavioral styles. These people often develop an impulsive style that leads them to be unaware of their impairments and causes them to wrongly assume that they can still perform the same tasks as before the stroke. This behavioral style can be extremely dangerous. It may lead the left hemiplegic stroke survivor to try to walk without aid. Or it may lead the survivor with spatial and perceptual impairments to try to drive a car (National Stroke Association, 1994, p.10).

Left-Hemisphere Stroke

The left hemisphere of the brain controls the movement of the right side of the body. It also controls speech and language abilities for most people.

A left-hemisphere stroke often causes paralysis of the right side of the body. This is known as *right hemiplegia*.

Someone who has had a left-hemisphere stroke may also develop *aphasia*. Aphasia is a catch-all term used to describe a wide range of speech and language problems. These problems can be highly specific, affecting only one component of the patient's ability to communicate, such as the ability to move their speech-related muscles to talk properly. The same patient may be relatively unimpaired when it comes to writing, reading, or under-standing speech.

People who have had a left-hemisphere stroke may develop memory problems similar to those of right-hemisphere stroke sur-vivors. These problems can include shortened retention spans, dif-ficulty in learning new information, and problems in conceptualiz-ing and generalizing. They may also have trouble with arithmetic.

Cerebellar Stroke

The cerebellum controls balance and coordination. A stroke that takes place in the cerebellum can cause coordination and bal-ance problems, dizziness, nausea and vomiting.

Brain Stem Stroke

Strokes that occur in the brain stem may be especially devas-tating. The brain stem is the area that controls all of our involun-tary, "life-support" functions, such as breathing, blood pressure, and heartbeat. The brain stem also controls abilities such as eye movements, hearing, well-articulated speech, and swallowing. Since impulses generated in the brain's hemispheres must travel through the brain stem on their way to the arms and legs, people who have had a brain stem stroke may also develop paralysis in one or both sides of the body.

Other Effects of Stroke

Finally, there are some general effects of stroke that seem to occur regardless of where in the brain the stroke took place. One of the most common of these is *emotional lability*, inappropriate laughter or crying that begins for no obvious reason and ends just as abruptly (National Stroke Association, 1994, pp. 11-12).

Further medical description, particularly the stroke physiology is discussed at length in Chapter 14.

Index